Disclaimer: Do not take this as medic~~al advice and always consult your~~ doctor (preferably a functional medi~~cal~~ program or diet. The author and tho~~se~~ responsible for any bullshit.

G000115729

Bullshit may or may not be limited mentally, or emotionally.

The stories and testimonies in this book are completely true and may or may not help you. God created each one of us different and unique with unique needs, so nothing is a one-size-fits-all answer. It may help; it may inspire; it may radically change your life, health, goals, family, joy, and marriage. It may not.

If you decide to undergo physical training and apply what I teach in this book, that is completely up to you and your physician and/or medical team. Reading this book does not make this a client-coach relationship between us, for each circumstance is different. What worked for me and my clients may or may not work for you.

There are many considerations to take in, such as injuries, medical conditions, a fully equipped gym, food allergies and intolerances, food sensitivities, metabolic syndrome, hormones, food uptake and absorption, gut health, mindset, believing in yourself, mind-muscle connection and control, deficiencies, and supplements, just to name a few.

Do not look at this as specific advice.

Take responsibility for your own actions whether you apply the content in this book or not. Be smart and be diligent in finding what is best for you and your journey.

If you get coffee, it may be hot. If you buy a bag of peanuts, it may have nuts. If you apply this book, you may have a transformed life.

Use what works for you. As my spiritual father Dr. John Watson told me years ago, "Eat the fish and spit out the bones."

Happy fishing!

THREE DAYS STRONG AF

THREE DAYS STRONG

AF

GET BUILT IN LESS TIME,
INCREASE YOUR ENERGY,
AND KICK ASS AT LIFE

BAILEY DAWN

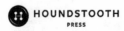
HOUNDSTOOTH
PRESS

THREE DAYS STRONG AF
Get Built in Less Time, Increase Your Energy, and Kick Ass at Life

FIRST EDITION

ISBN 978-1-5445-3859-4 *Hardcover*
978-1-5445-3860-0 *Paperback*
978-1-5445-3861-7 *Ebook*

This book is dedicated to my dad and coach, two legends I was honored and blessed to have in my life in becoming a high performer.

To Mike Bailey Sr.

Losing you took our world by surprise and heartache. You were a living example of strength and wisdom. You lived for your family and seeing smiles on our faces. My prayer is that others would read this book and become at least half the dad and husband you were. It wasn't fair the way you were taken from this world, but God still used you more than you ever realized. Even then you said, "Life isn't fair, but God is...and God is still good." You lived that.

I also used some cuss words on the cover and in a few places in this book. You might not like that, but that's a story for another day!

Thank you for teaching me how to do everything with my whole heart, for teaching me to love discipline and why, and how to be kind and gentle. Thank you for being so strong my whole life. You carried me like a baby when I learned how to walk again, and it was less than two years later you were bound to that same wheelchair that I knew too well. Thank you for teaching me how to curl a dumbbell when I was just five years old. Together, we climbed trees, caught so many critters and snakes, went on more road trips than any kid could dream of, and the best was seeing how well you cherished Mom and your faith. Thank you for teaching me to throw the ball harder than the other girls. I'm probably not allowed to say that, but you did.

You suffered more than anyone else I have ever known. But I've also learned that those who are the kindest were hurt the most. You were a beacon of light for every single person in your life. I was lucky enough to grow up and watch that with my own eyes, and it gave me a deeper perspective on writing this book.

To John Meadows,

Reading your eulogy was one of the hardest things I have ever done in my life. I looked into the eyes of your wife and twin twelve-year-old sons from the altar, sharing about your life and faith, and it's because of you I was able to write this book. So many people think they have to spend all their extra time in the gym while compromising relationships, but you showed me how far from the truth that was. You taught me a much better way and you took me under your wing.

Just two months after you passed, your boys won their football championship, and all I could see was you jumping, screaming, and celebrating them in heaven, so proud of them.

You took many people under your wing. People who became Olympians because of you. You changed the bodybuilding industry in the most positive way possible. It was more than just a sport to you. It was family.

Deep down, men desire to be just like you. They want success, respect, a happy family, good health, a loving marriage, and basically to be strong AF in every area of life just like you, all while still being present and full of joy and happiness. Of course, they don't have to be as large as your bodybuilding days but the lifestyle you lived. Even more importantly, deep down they need to be like you—humble, loving, loyal, and full of character.

You are forever a legend.

CONTENTS

CHAPTER 1

BECOMING A FIT OVERALL HIGH PERFORMER

At the age of fifty-eight, my dad had a bad reaction to a flu shot he was forced to get at work, and he was left paralyzed. My family and I watched in horror as his strong-like-an-ox, six-foot six-inch frame weakened, seemingly overnight. His broad shoulders sunk in, as if the muscles holding them up had disappeared. It looked like his collarbones had collapsed. After many tests, the doctor eventually said he didn't know what else to diagnose my dad with, so he called it amyotrophic lateral sclerosis, or ALS.

A fatal diagnosis with no hope.

The very words you never want to hear. A devastating diagnosis for anyone, but it felt especially cruel when applied to my father, a man who wanted to do so much more—to travel, to make more memories, to live.

We got that diagnosis two days after my fiancé proposed to me. My heart and mind were in a state of grief, not joy, but I wanted to bring some cheer to my family, so we went shopping for my wedding dress. I didn't even want to buy a dress that day; I simply hoped to see a smile on my dad's face.

As we drove to the dress shop, my dad sat in the passenger seat—he had already lost his ability to move his arms—and stared straight ahead through the windshield.

"I wish I had worked smarter and not harder," he said. He kept looking straight ahead.

I immediately had a flashback to reading *Rich Dad Poor Dad* by Robert Kiyosaki as a teenager. When I'd discussed the mindset of working smarter not harder with my dad back then, I only remember the look of disappointment on his face.

Dad worked hard and then harder. More and more hours. Even so, I grew up poor. We lived in a trailer park, and no matter how hard my dad worked, determined that we have class, we all struggled with that poverty mentality.

He worked two full-time jobs while serving the church and his community and was highly respected and loved by thousands of people—a bit of a local celebrity with tons of love to give. But when he was dying, he had a regret: that he hadn't worked smarter so he could have more time with the people he loved.

We got to the dress shop and I spun and twirled in a few wedding dresses. My dad seemed deep in thought. Then he smiled and told me I looked beautiful.

Within seven weeks of my dad's diagnosis, my fiancé and I had a small backyard ceremony. We were worried about whether he would even make it to that, but he was there, even though I basically carried him down the aisle because he could barely shuffle his feet. Even in that short amount of time, he had lost the ability to speak.

Even though he couldn't say it in words, I learned a valuable lesson from my dad: time waits on no one, no matter how hard you work.

THE GIFT OF TIME

What would you do with the gift of extra time?

Unfortunately, there is no such thing as extra time or creating time, for time is already set. We all have the same twenty-four hours in a day. And, in fact, we may have even less time than we think.

Let's break out some numbers here for this. (Note: these numbers are averages based on all people.)

- First you are born, and at that moment, statistically speaking, you have about seventy-eight years left.
- You are sleeping for about one-third of that time. That leaves you with about forty-nine waking years.
- You spend about 31,000 hours studying or in class to get educated. Added up, that's about three and a half years. You now have about forty-six years remaining.
- You spend (on average) 91,000 hours on your work. That's ten and a half years, with around thirty-five years left.
- The average person spends around one whole year in their car in traffic. Thirty-four.
- Brushing your teeth, sitting on the toilet, showering, and get-

ting ready takes off another two and a half years. You now have thirty-two years left.

- Eating and drinking takes four years. You have twenty-eight left.
- Shopping and grocery runs add up to about two and a half years. Cooking, cleaning, yard work, and other chores take about six years. Twenty years left.
- You spend a year and a half, total, caring for kids and loved ones. Eighteen precious years left...
- Of which you spend half watching TV, playing video games, or on Facebook. Or Reddit. Pick your poison; you spend nine years doing it. And that means you have nine years left.

Out of seventy-eight years on this earth, only nine are yours.[1]

Nine years to spend with your family and friends. To play, laugh, and cry. To fall in love. To see the world. To pursue your passions.

Are you still wasting your time on things that don't actually matter? Procrastinating on doing the things that matter most? Wasting more time in the gym than you need to?

What would you rather be doing?

Go do that instead.

Time is worth more than money. And when we get to the end of our lives, we will wish we had cherished it more instead of wasting it. A study was done for those at the end of their life, asking about

---

1   Gemma Curtis, "Your Life in Numbers," Sleep Matters Club, September 29, 2017, https://www. dreams.co.uk/sleep-matters-club/your-life-in-numbers-infographic/.

their regrets. Most of them wished they had spent their time with people they loved more and made more memories.

We will wish we had worked smarter, not harder. Not just with our careers but with our relationships, well-being, and fitness, too.

So break out of that cycle and live life to the fullest. Don't wait until you get the diagnosis or until you are at the end of your life—or even until your projects slow down.

There is more to life than hustling and busyness, but we often learn that too late. At the expense of our own health and well-being and at the expense of what really matters in life. At the expense of a failed marriage, shaky relationship with your kids, or dreams that have come and gone.

The beautiful thing is that it isn't too late to view time from a different perspective or to redefine success. To realize that perhaps you've been using the wrong measuring stick. It's okay to recalculate.

Do it before your health runs out. Do it before you shut down due to exhaustion. Do it before the greatest relationship of your life fades away. Do it before you miss out on your kids' recitals and baseball games.

You can have extreme results for your health and fitness in only three or four days a week, instead of spending more unnecessary time. If you can get the body you want in three hours a week instead of twelve, wouldn't you do it?

You'd get the body and health you want, plus save nine hours you can invest into other important areas of your life from your marriage, kids, hobbies, chasing some dreams, faith, and career.

What could you do with your marriage, family, health, and dreams if you had an extra nine hours?

This book can help you be healthy and fit without compromising the other areas of your life, such as your marriage, family, career, and dreams, and without wasting another extra minute of your time.

BUT WHO AM I?

I was raised to work hard. Growing up, I wanted to be the hardest working person in the room—and if I was, I needed to find a new room. I was raised to give 100 percent in everything I did, whether I was working at McDonald's, an athlete, or with patients.

When I was in high school, I became one of the fastest hurdlers in the state of Ohio, breaking records through my freshman year of college. At eighteen, I was the starting pitcher—and the only woman in the league—for an all-men's baseball team. By nineteen, I started volunteering, doing massage therapy for sports medicine physicians, physical therapists, and cancer patients.

Over the next twenty years, I became an entrepreneur, working my way to become a highly sought-after massage therapist who works with celebrities and professional athletes. During that time, I dedicated my twenties to more studies, traveling, ministry, and healing. By the age of thirty, I was competing in figure competitions and snowboarding at national levels. I became the team sports massage therapist for a major league soccer team.

After crushing my ankles while snowboarding on a pro tour (a story I'll share in a later chapter), I started bodybuilding.[2] I began winning most of the figure competitions I entered, finishing in the top ten nationally and top five in the amateur division of the Arnold Classic. After that, people asked me how I did it and what my training and nutrition secrets were. I started sharing that journey and coaching others along the way.

Ultimately, and with more than two decades of experience, I became a High Performance coach and author. More importantly, I am a wife and mom, and I desire more of God. I keep the important things most important. That was another beautiful lesson my dad taught me.

I am obsessed with becoming my best in every area of life while remaining balanced and confident. This means simplifying my training and nutrition to be as healthy and fit as I want. I don't have to be in the gym every day to stay fit, and by not spending all my time there, I am able to perform higher in all the other areas of my life.

Years ago, I decided I wanted to learn more about training and nutrition. I went the most effective way and worked with the professional that bodybuilding magazines interviewed and who professional wrestlers and NFL players hired. I didn't want to eat like a rabbit or run on a treadmill like a damn hamster to get results like most trainers had me do.

I wanted to know what the best of the best were doing, so I contacted John Meadows.[3] He was not only successful with his

---

2   There are different categories in the sport of bodybuilding, such as bikini, physique, fitness, figure, wellness, and bodybuilding itself. Each category has specific features and poses that the judges look for.

3   Mountain Dog Diet, accessed September 20, 2022, https://mountaindogdiet.com/.

bodybuilding career and his physique but also as a business owner, devoted husband, and father. His marriage, family, faith, and career were not on the back burner to be in the professional shape that he was in.

After I wrote this book, I was told, with great sadness, that John passed unexpectedly and peacefully in his sleep due to a suspected pulmonary embolism. The fitness industry and bodybuilding community worldwide he left behind still mourns the hole in our hearts. Yet I hope that, while you are reading, he can inspire you as he has inspired me and so many others—and, in fact, he is the inspiration for this entire book.

There are many fitness influencers and coaches, but we are not all the same. What makes this book completely different from the rest is the focus on becoming an overall higher performer while getting in the shape of your dreams. You don't have to train like an athlete, but you can learn from the professionals.

I wrote this book because I was using less time in the gym than everyone else but getting on stage and winning competitions without using fat burners and without any type of drug, hormone blocker, or enhancer. If anything, I have a hormone issue that makes it even more difficult to get ripped and easier to hold body fat. People were asking me what I ate and how I trained to compete the way I did.

So that's what my training and nutrition program is—it's exactly what I did and do to be as strong and lean as I want to be in minimal time so I can focus on the high-performing life that I describe. You can have the life you want while still having the health and body you want, too.

I've used this program to win shows. It's more than just lift this or eat that, but it comes down to your mindset and your beliefs. It's more mental training than physical training.

You are able to train your mind to move toward your goals while keeping your health and family a priority. There's no need to be in the gym six to seven days a week and counting every blasted calorie if you can put your energy to doing it right.

In this book, I've simplified everything I have learned as a competitor, therapist, and coach to make it more straightforward and more useful. I've taken out all the extra fluff so you can get straight to the health and body you want, and so you can become a high performer, too!

WHAT DO I MEAN BY HIGH PERFORMER?

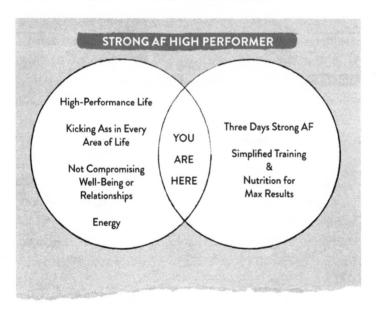

STRONG AF HIGH PERFORMER

High-Performance Life

Kicking Ass in Every Area of Life

YOU ARE HERE

Three Days Strong AF

Simplified Training & Nutrition for Max Results

Not Compromising Well-Being or Relationships

Energy

I bet you are wondering what a high performer is. Well, first, it's a term I love (and it was coined by Brendon Burchard, to give credit where credit is due), and it's used to describe pretty much my most favorite people in the world.

High performers aren't just people who are successful, rich, and famous, so scrap that from your mind right now. A high performer can be anyone who sustains long-term success. From professional athletes, CEOs, students, Uber drivers, to hair stylists. Literally anyone in any field, sustaining long-term success without compromising well-being or relationships, is a high performer.

High performers have the most robust conversations yet remain balanced. They seek to be successful on a long-term basis, so it's sustainable. And they don't have a "hustling" mindset, like you might think.

Hustling 24/7 can pretty much kill you and your success if you don't find a way to get some balance into your life. In all the time I've worked with high performers, I've seen the mindsets, lives, failures, successes, what works, and what doesn't. I've seen the pain and misery of those who strive and strive and strive and hustle and hustle and obsess and obsess to the point of literally breaking down their own health, marriage, and family.

They become the most isolated, lonely, and miserable people. By hustling and chasing success, they lose sight of things that are truly the most important in life, and ultimately kill their happiness by chasing the misconception of what success really is. (Ah, happiness. That can't be chased either or else you'll end up miserable, too.)

I work with a millionaire named Daniel who believes in the old-school hustler mentality. He's so focused on the money that he sits at his desk all day and sometimes all night working. Hustling isn't the answer like he thinks because even though he has the money, he's also had multiple joint replacements at too young an age from refusing to change.

"Rest is for the dead," he says.

No! That old-school thinking is damaging at the expense of your own time, health, and relationships.

Daniel would probably make even more money and make a greater impact and achieve greater overall success if he thought outside the box of just working harder. Most of us would. Imagine what you could be capable of by working smarter and allowing your mind to be renewed and even more productive because of it.

See, that's part of what makes a true high performer different than the rest. It's more than just making money and working yourself to death; it's someone who can be successful for a long period of time while having a great well-being and relationships. A high performer is overall more successful in whatever field they are in. They are genuinely happier, too. They have better relationships with their spouses.

A high performer isn't someone who is just kicking ass in one area of life, while all the other areas are crumbling and suffering, but they advance in all areas (relationally, emotionally, mentally, physically) and are able to sustain it.

Imagine the life of bringing it all together for your happiness, health, and even making better money doing what you love.

Sounds like they're pretty successful, right? I think so! But it all depends on your definition of success.

BUT FIRST, LET'S REDEFINE SUCCESS

Mr. Banks was an established man in London and very focused on his work. It seemed his relationship with his wife had dwindled down to tasks to run an orderly home and to hire a full-time nanny to raise his children with discipline.

Then Mary Poppins came to the rescue.

I'm sure you are familiar with the classic story. Mr. Banks was so focused on the shiny distraction of becoming what he thought was successful. Even though he did it for the children, it was the children who were hurting and his wife who was always trying to mend the pieces. At the end of the movie, he finally realized what true success was and redirected his vision and purpose.

Don't wait until the end of your movie to redirect and redefine your success. Start today.

Let's look at setting yourself up for success...true success.

The definition of true success can look different for each person, but it begins with the mindset of a high performer.

A lot of people look successful on the outside with money and power, but in the long run, they are miserable and corrupt. That's not the kind of success you want to aim for, no matter how shiny and glamorous it seems. There is more to success than just money and jets. Yes, you can have those things, but that is not what defines success, nor how to get there.

So it's not just money and power and a luxurious life that makes you a successful high performer. You can start from where you are, in any field, and from any demographic and just be consistent with what I'm about to teach you.

It's about creating a high-performance life in which you experience ongoing joy, engagement, and confidence from being your best self without destroying your health and relationships to get there. It's how you master your mind and body for lasting change and success.

It begins in your mind and it takes some practice, which I'll go over in this book. As you master your mind and body, you can master your success with the tools I have laid out for you. You can be the much happier version of Mr. Banks but with your dream body.

This book not only helps you to redefine success, but it helps you to master your mind and body to make it last. You get the success you want, plus being in the best shape of your life, and the tools that show you exactly how to do it and maintain it.

You can get any kind of productivity tool, diet, workout, and information for free off the internet.

What you can't get is how to master your mind and body with it, and that's why this book is uniquely different.

You can become more of the person you want to become.

HOW TO BE A SUCCESSFUL HIGH PERFORMER AND GET IN THE BEST SHAPE OF YOUR LIFE

High performers want it all. They want to excel at everything that matters and not waste time on what doesn't. They are uniquely productive and do what matters most in life.

They want to be healthy, strong, lean, and feel confident going to the gym. They want an awesome workout to get the best results in minimal time and to keep succeeding in all the other areas, too.

Performing well in all areas of your life including getting ripped, without killing what matters most, is how you get the transformation you want in the most effective way. This allows you to easily plan time in the gym, lift hard, know how to fuel yourself well, and head out to do well in the other areas with work and family.

Imagine simplifying your training and nutrition to only three days a week. This way, you can have four out of the seven days away from the gym to work with hawklike focus on projects, time to rejuvenate your mind and soul, and time to engage and connect with the people you love. Shoot, maybe you can even pick up that new hobby if you wanted.

My goal for you is to really get into your head to realize how to work out and eat so you can go from a high performer to an even higher performer.

You don't want to get to the end of your life and realize that you didn't get to see what you were truly made of because you were too busy doing the unessential things. You were too busy being busy that you missed out on the important things.

You don't want to end up like Daniel hustling his life and joints into the ground, with no joy or health. You don't want to be Mr. Banks for your whole life (but at least he redirected and discovered joy in his life again).

By applying what I show you, it will allow room for your mindset to grow, and your perspective can shift in a positive way. Like Mary Poppins to Mr. Banks, except this Mary Poppins gets you jacked in the gym. By following my program, you can get ripped, but do it more effectively in half the time, which will lead to deeper relationships, being healthier and more fit, and having more confidence and increased joy.

DEEPER RELATIONSHIPS

After years of being in the fitness industry and as a wellness expert, I've seen many marriages and families fall apart because of obsession and addiction to be in competitive shape. People obsess over every calorie they eat, and they work out more hours than needed and avoid where time is needed most.

What if you could have that healthy and fit body in the most effective time so you can be more present in the relationships that matter most to you? You can still get in the best shape of your life without obsessing about every calorie and being in the gym five or six days a week.

You aren't worried about calculating macros; not freaking out because of the never-ending list of tasks and projects; not stressed out like usual, because you are learning how to create healthier boundaries. You're also learning how to take better care of yourself and those around you who need you on your A game.

We are wired and created for healthy relationships, so we need to learn to contribute to them. Like a garden, relationships won't thrive if left unattended.

HEALTHIER AND MORE RIPPED

There's no easy way around this one, but most high performers want to be healthy and have their best physique. Your health is often put on the back burner to meet deadlines or when life is stressful. However, one major thing that a fixed mindset needs to change is neglecting your health.

So if you want to be healthier or to have that lean and built physique, be more assertive with yourself to make this possible. You are a high performer. That means you will always have deadlines and projects to do, but your health should never be last.

When setting yourself up for this success, your health will help you perform even better overall.

When you feel better, you are healthier, sleeping better, drinking more water, more aware, more present, enjoying life, have quality and deep relationships, happier, in the best shape of your life, and perform better at home and work.

When you are healthier, you set yourself up for success.

The most productive people make time for their health, and the top 5 percent of the highest performers around the world exercise three days a week. When you think and live your life in an essential way, that does what matters most, you become more effective with your time. This includes how to get healthy and ripped in the most effective amount of time.

High performers do not re-create the wheel and make it harder on themselves, and neither should you.

GREATER CONFIDENCE

It's important that we really drive home the importance of mindset for a forever-changed result to get the life, health, and body you want. If you are looking for some silly fad diet or get-skinny formula, then put this book down right now and walk away.

This book is for high performers who want to perform higher in all areas of life. I've condensed the training and nutrition from the most experienced bodybuilders and self-care rituals of professional athletes to make it most effective, so you are not wasting time in the gym like that hamster on a wheel with no purpose.

You can no longer waste time. Instead, use this guide to get you the results you want in less time. You'll walk into the gym with more confidence because you have a plan...not a hamster wheel and rabbit food.

JOY, NOT JUST HAPPINESS

Happiness is a dead end. I see and hear people chasing it all the time, and part of me wonders, "So did you catch it yet?"

Happiness is a choice, not a destination or achievement. Choose happiness; don't chase it. It's not about waiting for the new deal, the new promotion, winning the lottery, going on that dream vacation, or marrying your best friend and having perfect kids that will give you happiness. That may make you happy for a moment, but at some point you have to come back to reality and go back to chasing your next "happiness fix."

It turns into an addiction.

A selfish one.

Is there anything wrong with being happy? Absolutely not, but it's the mindset toward it that really messes with people's lives to where they simply don't find happiness.

Joy, however, is something else to have your heart and mind focused on.

It's deeper than happiness. Happiness is fleeting. Happiness is something you can choose to be no matter your circumstance.

But joy—that's deep. It's more than just a feeling. It radiates through every part of you.

Joy is found on the other side of hard work and sometimes suffering.

Becoming a high performer will help you experience more joy by learning how to kick ass in every area of your life. Not just by getting built and being obsessed about it but having a more holistic approach to your overall well-being. Each week, you will begin to evaluate how much joy you are experiencing, and you'll make goals to increase that joy.

Recently, I met up with a dear friend for scotch and cigars. We slid our Don Pepin cigars from their plastic sleeves, struggled to cut the ends with a dull cutter, and took turns lighting our cigars.

We puffed, sipping on our scotch and savoring the moment.

The conversation turned toward how we were recovering and praying through hard moments in life, for ourselves and those whom we love. Michael said, "Sadness and joy are brother and sister. You can't have joy without sadness. And you can't understand or appreciate either without the other."

It's important to feel, examine oneself, and be present. It's one thing to choose happiness, but you've got to be willing to sit with sadness before truly experiencing joy.

High performers don't chase happiness; they pursue joy.

WHAT DOES LIFE LOOK LIKE AS A HIGH PERFORMER?

You are either already a high performer or taking your steps to become one.

You know there is more to life than black and white, fat checks, and pretending like you have it all together. You don't want to trade your spouse in like a car for the newer updated model. You don't want to invite trauma to your kids. You don't want to work yourself to death while forgetting about your own well-being. Don't fall for the misconception of what some think success is. Instead, take the higher road that begins with mastering your mind and body with the mindset of a high performer.

When you are a high performer, you want to move forward in all areas of life. You want to have a more productive mind; you're open to more opportunities and experiences; and you cut out what isn't essential to you or your goals.

You aren't always on overdrive anymore. No longer on the road to exhaustion and burnout, but you learn how to balance it. You aren't waiting until things slow down or you hit your numbers in order to take care of the more important things in life.

You no longer put your own health and happiness on the back burner. You even learn something greater than happiness—that's called joy—and what that looks like and feels like.

You have a fulfilled relationship and look forward to growing old together and sharing life together, cheering each other on.

You are no longer wasting your time that could be invested in doing something so much more profitable for you. You invest in places of finances, faith, well-being, overall health, joy, personal development, community, and of course, relationships. You can't invest into everything, but discover where you can.

You get the health and body you want, and you don't have to kill yourself in the gym and starve yourself to get it. You want to see what you're made of as a high performer and to continue growing and performing higher.

You are able to do more because you've learned what is essential in life, what is distracting, and how to manage your time to get the most out of it. You do it without compromising well-being and relationships, becoming overall happier, healthier, and more successful. You gain more, yet find yourself doing less, so you can appreciate more and enjoy your life more. You don't have regrets at the end of your life.

You aren't so busy anymore, and you can actually think straight compared to what you used to do. Instead, you have boundaries that line up with the direction you are going. If it's not a hell yes, it should be a hell no.

You are healthy and fit. You didn't wait for an ultimate health scare to get there. You keep your health a priority and see how it negatively affects your productivity and overall happiness if you don't. You understand the importance of prevention and not just waiting for things to go wrong.

You pursue your spouse for years to come and never stop dating each other and having fun. You find ways to keep it fun and fresh. You grow old together despite all the younger, flashier models out there who want to steal your attention. I know because for many years, I was asked to be that younger model.

Your kids see the way you love and respect each other, and they grow up to marry someone who loves them as much as you two do. Your kids grew up to see how you used each day to make it a better place or a better family, so they learned from you and grew to multiply what you modeled for them. Isn't that a success to aspire to achieve?

You continue to nurture positive relationships in your life, finding ways to serve your community, and making an impact.

You have control over your finances and budget, feeling joy because of how much you can bless others with your generosity with time and money in ways you never thought you could.

Your life as a high performer is not only for you but how much more you can impact the world and your family. It becomes your legacy.

You are capable of all this, but it's up to you to believe it, envision it, and even to define your own success and what that means to you. You are living and breathing what success really is.

Maybe all you care about is being rich and having your own island. But what good is it to be alone on it or stuck on it with a frail or fleeting relationship? Or all the extra work and stress you just signed up for to maintain your island? But hey, you have an island. Great job, I guess, but this book isn't for you unless you want more for your life and those you share it with.

It may sound daunting to some to feel like you must achieve all those things. Heck, it might stress you out just thinking about it, and it might make you not want to try.

How about you try to envision what your future looks like and feels like? Are you alone and just making money? Are you in a mutually supportive marriage and look forward to date nights, while also performing well in your career or business?

You feel love, healthy, happiness, joy, security, brilliant, balanced, all while performing higher.

So yes, you really can have clear goals, manage time better, become more productive, accomplish more, do less, have deeper relationships, be healthy, smart, and fit. People live that life every day. It's a matter of practicing what those have mastered already, like John Meadows. Even then, there is still always room to grow and fine-tune.

It may take some practice to do it all well, but it's about practice.

Do you think professional athletes just magically make those miracle ESPN highlight catches without practice? That one World Series game-saving catch probably took twelve years of consistent practice, to only be seen once by everyone else when it mattered the most.

Well, your life matters. Your relationships matter. Your joy matters. Your health and fitness matter! Your success matters! Your growth matters! It all matters. You keep practicing it every damn day, not to be seen but still do it as if it were. Practice like it matters.

And reading this book is your practice.

I have intentionally broken this book into three parts. In Part I, you will learn how having the mindset of a high performer will help you find true success. In Part II, we will focus on how nutrition can help you get in better shape faster. In Part III, you'll see how weightlifting brings it all together, and I'll give you workout tips for all levels, from beginners to elite athletes.

Now that I'm in your head on what success could be like for you as a high performer, we will do exercises that take it into your heart to practice every day. Then you can make your own World Series game-saving catch and have your own ESPN highlight.

JUMP IN!

You know, the people who get the farthest in life are the ones who are willing to jump in and to completely immerse themselves.

I only want good things for you; I promise you that. I'm here to teach you, guide you, challenge you, propel you, and give you everything that I practice and the highest performers from around the world practice.

So come hungry, absorb, immerse, engage as much as possible. Don't just be a wallflower watching everybody else; engage and immerse. Do the exercises I give you; don't just listen. If you want to get the most out of this book, then put in as much as you want to get out.

Wallflowers don't get anywhere but depressed. If that's you, then pry yourself from the wall and dance anyway. You can't hide in the corner and cry because nobody is asking you to dance. This whole life is your dance; don't wait for someone else to ask you.

Dance.

Don't wait on others to make it happen. The power is yours, and it's always been yours.

It's like some people hire a trainer but don't actually do the workouts or make the diet changes. It's not the trainer's fault, sweetheart; but we both knew that.

Don't make it harder on yourself, but instead set yourself up for lasting success.

There is no dabbling or just trying it out to see if it works. Just so you know, those people never get anywhere near as far as the ones who immerse themselves, and I don't want you to settle, but I can't force you.

If you want to get somewhere, you have to commit and completely immerse yourself.

Are you ready? Let's dive in!

KEY TAKEAWAY

Becoming a high performer is more than just sitting around and talking about it.

It's more than just being super fit. It's more than just being awesome at your job or business. It's habits so you can continuously succeed for a long period of time without compromising your wellbeing or relationships. It's actually a more holistic and balanced approach, so you are able to focus more, become more successful and productive, get more done, be less busy, be more fulfilled, happier, healthier, and more engaged.

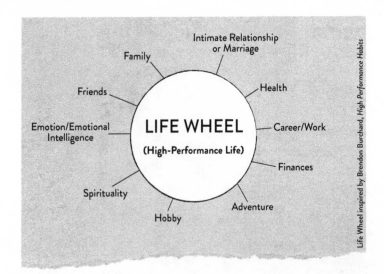

LIFE WHEEL
(High-Performance Life)

Intimate Relationship or Marriage
Family
Friends
Health
Emotion/Emotional Intelligence
Career/Work
Finances
Spirituality
Adventure
Hobby

Life Wheel inspired by Brendon Burchard, *High Performance Habits*

HIGH-PERFORMANCE EXERCISE

I want you to have a more holistic view of your life, starting today. Organize your life into ten categories: health, family, friends, intimate relationship, mission/work, finances, adventure, hobby, spirituality, and emotion. These ten categories originally appeared in Brendon Burchard's *High Performance Habits*, but I like to call them your life wheel.

Once you have those ten categories written down, rate your level of joy in each area on a scale of one to ten, and write your goals in each of these ten areas every weekend.

It's a very valuable way to measure your life and become more aware. If you don't, then you won't know how to balance things, measure them, or become more successful with them.

So right now, on a piece of paper, write down those ten areas and rate them.

Make goals in each to increase your joy and mastering your mind and body to lasting change and success.

1. After completing your life wheel with rating and goals, visualize your goals and who you want to be. What does that life look like to you? How do you feel? Are you feeling happy, healthy, connected, driven, successful? Close your eyes and take this exercise seriously. Try to feel how you want to feel. *Feel the feels.* Write them down.

2. One-Year-from-Now Exercise: In each area, write down the date one year from now and look back on what you have accomplished, as if you are one year in the future and looking back to today. What progress have you made over the past year? How can you make the next year look like the year you have envisioned?

    a. Marriage on the rocks and want to be happy again? Be honest to your spouse about couples coaching and counseling to deepen your relationship instead of allowing it to drift further apart.

    b. Is your career goal to become indispensable and valuable beyond measure? Starting your own business? Hiring a team, personal development, becoming more productive?

    c. What about your health goals? Are you a runner? Lifting weights? Outdoors hiking or snowboarding? Are you feeling good with being vegan, paleo, or completely cutting out the pop? Do you feel strong? Flexible? Getting regular massages, planning retreats, and self-care?

4. Go through each one. Really paint a picture of what you want to feel. Write it down and put it on your wall/mirror/screensaver to visualize and meditate on every single day.

5. If you wanted to get in the best shape of your life this year, when will you start and what would that look like?

6. What obstacles do you need to overcome in order to start and commit?

7. Are you willing to commit to your health and fitness? Will you make the changes you need to make?

PART I

MINDSET

When I was a young, brand-new massage therapist, building my clientele and struggling to pay bills, I worked full time for spas and physicians. I was on call for five-star hotels. Guests would come into town and schedule a massage with the concierge. Then I would bring all of my equipment, set it up at the hotel, and give the guest the best professional massage I possibly could. (Nothing dirty; don't let your mind go there!)

Sometimes I met celebrities who gave me tickets to their concerts and games and offered to fly me around the world. Most of the time, though, I didn't even know until afterward that I had just worked with someone famous. The concierge would say, "Bailey, do you have any idea who you were just talking to?" I was clueless. Celebrities want to be treated like a normal person anyway, so it helped that I didn't know who they were unless they were LeBron James or the Rock.

Regardless if a client was a celebrity or not, I had one simple rule for every deep tissue massage I gave: give them the best massage they have ever had. One person told me, "Wow! I've had massages from Madonna's therapist, and yours are even better!" Each time, my goal was to give them a massage that was better than the one before, which forced me to perform higher as a therapist and as a listener.

One celebrity flew to my city on a regular basis for his massages. He asked me to be his full-time massage therapist and offered to pay me full time plus travel. He wanted to fly me around the world on his personal jet, inviting me to stay in his many homes and talked of some private island. He also promised to introduce me to other celebrities on the island.

Wow! A celebrity inviting me to meet more celebrities! I couldn't believe it. It seemed like a dream come true. This would be the perfect opportunity to meet and work with successful people around the world and get better at my craft.

I was on cloud nine.

Until the next appointment went terribly wrong. I learned he wanted me to do more than massage. I hid in the hotel bathroom after he reached for himself under the linens and began masturbating. He didn't want a therapist; he wanted to groom me for sexual acts.

His personal assistants continued to call and harass me, wanting me to accept his offer. I was informed multiple times how large his penis was, how rich he was, and how many homes he had. But I knew that no amount of success was worth forfeiting my self-respect.

I changed my phone number and never looked back.

THIS IS NOT SUCCESS

Unfortunately, that wasn't the last time something like that happened.

Another powerful man with lots of money and influence came to me for regular massages. He learned that I had dreams to be in the next Winter Olympics in snowboarding. However, the equipment, traveling, training, coaches, and fees were expensive, so I couldn't afford it.

He offered to sponsor me and pay for everything, saying, "I believe in your dreams, and I want to see you reach them."

My dreams.

Everything.

Right in front of me.

I choked back tears so he couldn't see them in the dim light of the massage room. I was thinking, *This is it! My dreams of being an Olympian are going to come true!* I knew I had a long way to go, but I was willing to do whatever it took to live my dream.

Until I realized just what that price was.

Just like the dirty celebrity with a fancy jet, this man—who was married to his wife of twenty years and who had two kids—wanted me to be the lady on the side and lower my self-worth. It made me sick and left me wondering, *Is this what it takes to be successful?*

So far, I was learning that success wasn't about hard work, focusing on goals, and mastering my sport. Instead, these corrupt men wanted me to think that success came only as a result of disrespecting myself and sleeping around.

No dream is worth that. Needless to say, I cut all ties with that sponsor.

I thought it was my fault that I was attracting these dirtbags, so I began to wear baggy Thai pants that I had to wrap around me twice and tie with a rope, with a baggy shirt, and I hid under a baseball cap. Even with these outward protections, similar things happened for twenty years.

Fitness photographers would ask to photograph me for their portfolio, but when I looked into their portfolios, it was more like porn. I didn't train this hard to be in porn.

I declined every time someone made me one of those offers. Through those experiences, I learned what success is.

It's not about being rich, powerful, or having your own private jet.

Instead, true success is having the habits and the mindset of a high performer.

CHAPTER 2

LEARN FROM PROFESSIONAL ATHLETES WHY MINDSET AND SELF-CARE IS CRUCIAL TO YOUR OVERALL PERFORMANCE

My client Blayne was feeling defeated after taking a hard hit to the head. He had a pretty bad concussion—enough for him to need a few months of regular appointments with a neurologist.

He was on my table in the training room, which was closely packed with other players around us doing their specific therapies. One player balanced on one leg on a movable Bosu ball, post knee surgery to work on stability, while kicking the ball at the same time. Other guys took turns in the three different ice baths.

Blayne laid faceup on the table waiting for me to work on his muscles. I brought out a tiny bottle of pure frankincense oil to use around the occipital area. With a few drops on the palms of my hands, I guided Blayne through deep breathing techniques to muffle out the noise around us. My hands hovered over his eyes and nose to help calm him, and he inhaled the aromatherapy while lowering his shoulders away from his ears. I used my thumbs to find trigger points that help with headaches and tension release through his skull, neck, and trapezius muscles. He breathed deeply and sighed with relief as if nothing else was going on around us.

Because of his brain injury, it was more important than ever for Blayne to be proactive, to heal, and not push through anything. He had to take more steps back than he ever wanted, right at the height of his career. Faith, patience, and mindfulness helped his mind heal in this downtime.

We celebrated the moment his doctor cleared him to be on field again.

However, we soon moaned and groaned with him when a fellow teammate took a knee to the back of Blayne's head, giving him another brain injury. That meant another few months out, costing him a big chunk of the season.

But after more time of healing and focusing on his faith, recovery, and rest, he came out stronger. In fact, he was invited as the team captain for the United States National Team.

If he wouldn't have respected those brain injuries and the time needed to heal, he wouldn't have landed where he was so powerfully. That time off taught him more than what he expected, although it was difficult to do.

Blayne says, "I think the time off put so much into perspective in terms of what I love about my career and job. It revealed how much I love what I do, and how difficult it is to be away from it. But more importantly, it taught me how patience is an undeniable virtue. Gather as much information as you can about your issues and then trust the process of rehabilitation. Not easy but it got me on the other side with a healthy brain and a better outlook on life and soccer."

THE IMPORTANCE OF MINDSET AND SELF-CARE

Blayne's story is important because it shows how mindset and overall self-care is crucial to your performance. The more you adopt the mindset and overall self-care like Blayne, the better you can perform. Not just as an athlete but as a high performer.

Another time, my massage table was set up in the middle of the training room where the MLS players filtered in for their treatment after training. Their recovery process was just as important as the training process. That's why professional athletes heal faster than average people. They go through intense training, games, and get right back on the field or court. Without the best treatment, they wouldn't play as well.

When the soccer players came off the field, they showered and immediately came into the training room for medical treatment to get them right back on the field. This meant specialized strength and conditioning to correct imbalances, ice packs, ice baths, electrical stimulation, ultrasound, massage, compression wraps, and many other methods that were personalized for each player's needs.

Without this kind of self-care and medical treatment, they wouldn't always be able to get back in the game, nor be at the top of their game. They would be out longer with injuries and that would invite even more injuries. Think of the medical team like self-care. Without it, they wouldn't be able to perform and recover at their best.

This is why weekend warriors and amateur athletes have more injuries; they simply don't give themselves the same care. Whether they don't have it or seek it out, it's part of why they have the most injuries.

But this concept isn't just for athletes. If you want to perform well, then it is a must to make self-care part of your performance plan. It's your treatment to get back in the game, stay in the game, and succeed well for a long time.

By accepting this mindset transfer deposit, you are choosing the importance of self-care as part of your performance plan. If you want to go far and perform well, self-care is part of it. Think of it as recovery. Think of it as rejuvenating your mind.

Without it, you are running on exhaustion, injuries, and overwhelm. No room for longevity.

Maybe you don't have a medical team surrounding you each day, but there are still some valuable lessons to learn from them about how mindset and overall self-care is crucial to performance.

Performing well is more than just hustling hard every day. At some point, that hustler lifestyle is not sustainable and in fact, it can knock you back with health problems, depression, anxiety, and loneliness.

In the last chapter, we covered how to define success and what that looks like to you. Now we'll talk about all that's involved to get that success and stay there, and the treatment it takes to perform over and over again. You need that treatment to perform your best, to succeed, and to be fit and healthy. Professional athletes didn't accidentally become that way, nor will your success come accidentally.

This applies to your entrepreneurial goals, health goals, relationship goals, and anything else as you work toward your success. You don't just want to play the game, but you want to do your best so you can be your best, be successful, be confident, be healthy, be fit, and overall be happier, too.

HEALING AND POWER OF THE MIND

When I am in massage sessions with clients who have extremely stressful demands, one aspect of the session is mental. For however minutes they have hired me to heal them, we focus on the mind having a break. A break from thinking about solutions, deadlines, stresses, in-laws, and whatever other pains they are dealing with.

I've worked on countless athletes. One NFL player would come in for a regular session to get everything practically pounded out of him, but then one session was different. He was under a lot of stress from family pressures taking advantage of him, his money, and his success.

He had a look of defeat and exhaustion over him like I've never seen in him before and said, "I just want to relax and be somewhere else in my mind today."

We focused on meditation, deep breathing exercises, and prayer and changed the intense pressure he normally likes to something a little bit more blended to help him relax mentally. I blended deep tissue, trigger point, and sports massage, with moments of soothing restoration and relaxation. We were able to walk through guided meditation exercises to walk away from the stress and pressures temporarily and give his mind and emotions time to be restored.

When we were done, he said, "That was the best massage I have ever, ever gotten. Wow. I thought I just needed to be beat up and fixed every time, but I've never been here mentally before."

When you are pounded and just hustling hard all the time and trying to perform under exhaustion, your life and success is going to suffer somewhere. You need to allow time to be renewed mentally and physically. People try to perform under this pressure and exhaustion for too long and it often hurts them. To perform higher like successful high performers do, then renewal, restoration, and recovery is crucial to success.

Being able to walk away from constant pressure or hustling allows time for the mind and body to heal. Even this NFL player thought he needed to be physically pounded for all of his massage therapy sessions in order to improve. He came from the old-school mentality of "no pain, no gain." We still use deep tissue techniques, but it's blended with relaxation techniques to benefit his mind.

Imagine living your life with that approach. Imagine giving your mind permission to go somewhere else so you can relax, heal, escape from pressure, and have a fresh perspective. It increases your productivity when you come back. It's like hitting the reset button.

When faced constantly with stress without a place to find refuge in, the brain cannot heal and rejuvenate. The brain can adjust to pressure; however, to perform at your best for a sustainable amount of time to be a higher performer, rest and self-care must be part of your life on a regular basis. If not, you'll be ragged, exhausted, burned out, with joint replacements and many other health issues.

When allowing time to heal, that's when the mind is being replenished, refueled, rested, and rejuvenated to get back out in whatever game you are playing. You'll be in a better place mentally and physically. Not just as an athlete, but to take that athlete mentality to place into your own game as the high performer you are.

If you desire success, happiness, and health, you just can't achieve that and keep it for very long with the old-school hustler attitude. You'll find yourself trapped there. If you want to succeed, it's up to you to make it happen.

HOW YOUR MINDSET TRAINING CAN CREATE LASTING MENTAL, EMOTIONAL, AND PHYSICAL CHANGE

Be resilient as you become a higher performer. Decide what you want and what you don't want; decide it every single day. Meditate on it; write it down.

So the question is, what kind of higher performer do you want to be, and what does your life look like? What does it feel like? What kind of goals do you have? What do you not want to do or what do you not want to be?

When you can visualize it and dream it, then you can put it into action. Olympians don't just show up and perform well; they visualize it and meditate on it. They perform it over and over again in their mind so when it comes to show time, it appears they've done it effortlessly.

Translate this same mental skill into your physical training to get even better results. Make the changes you have always wanted to make, but now you can do it in less time so you can perform even higher in all the other areas you are visualizing.

Russian scientists compared four groups of Olympic athletes in terms of their training schedules:

- Group one had 100 percent physical training.
- Group two had 75 percent physical training with 25 percent mental training.
- Group three had 50 percent physical training with 50 percent mental training.
- Group four had 25 percent physical training with 75 percent mental training.

The results showed that group four, with 75 percent of their time devoted to mental training, performed the best. They have discovered the importance of mental strength before physical strength.

Let me tell you, it was not done effortlessly. It was a lifetime of training their minds and then their bodies followed. It's training their subconscious mind to move toward their plan, and you can, too.

Every single morning before you reach for your phone, begin training your mind with everything you just visualized for yourself. Start your day off right and finish it strong, because how you spend your day is how you spend your life.

Remember that only nine years are really yours to do with what you want.

ATHLETE PRACTICES TO APPLY TO YOUR OWN PERFORMANCE AND RECOVERY

TREATMENT LIKE A PRO

Describe your health and fitness goals.

List prevention techniques like a pro (weekly massages, nutrition, correction exercises, meditation, etc.).

What is an ideal schedule for you to practice the above to perform your best and actively prevent problems?

How would being healthier, pain-free, stronger, and leaner impact your life, energy, and career?

Begin a time and money budget to make these happen for you.
Add to your One Year from Now.

Here are some best practices used by athletes that you can apply to your own performance and recovery.

THINK PREVENTATIVELY

Instead of waiting for pain, injury, burnout, health problems, or until your marriage fades, put plans into action with your doctor to stay on top of things.

LACROSSE BALLS

The majority of my clients hold tension in their traps and between their shoulder blades. A lacrosse ball is the perfect material to do self-massage and dig out some trigger points and tension. This is great to use between your massage and chiropractic appointments.

MASSAGE THERAPY

Just like any career, a good therapist is rare to find! Generally, getting one massage a month is very helpful to your physical and mental health, but each person responds to stress and massage differently. I see many people on a weekly basis because it's that beneficial to their recovery and performance, while some only come when they want something fixed.

CHIROPRACTOR

I absolutely love chiropractors and a good adjustment! So often, pains that we have from stress, overuse, or poor posture can be helped or even prevented through an adjustment. I personally get adjusted once a month and sometimes more.

PHYSICAL THERAPIST

Really good ones are hard to find. Although many people can get the relief they need through massage and chiropractic, the problem often comes back until the original problem is corrected. A really good PT can see which muscles are being activated more than others and where some muscles aren't firing at all, causing all sorts of imbalances. Think of this like a circus tent with many poles. An imbalance is like having a pole lying on the ground and wondering why one section of the tent is caving in. The pole needs to be corrected, and a good therapist can help you train your mind to retrain your body to activate the correct muscles.

FUNCTIONAL MEDICINE DOCTORS

They see what traditional doctors don't. Although I go to traditional doctors for emergency situations, functional medicine go directly to the root and focuses on true health. They look at healing the person and look at things from a cellular level that most physicians would overlook. This particular doctor saved my life when a traditionally trained MD couldn't.

HEAT AND ICE TREATMENTS

Most of the MLS players were using ice treatment and walking away with ice bags wrapped around their injuries. There are healing benefits to using both heat and ice. By using wraps with Velcro, we can easily wrap heat or ice as needed to increase healing and decrease swelling. However, as DPT Corey Southers shared, the best is using heat from within your own body with specific movements, unless it's an acute injury.[4]

NUTRITION

Professional athletes use nutrition to properly fuel their minds and bodies. Although many registered dietitians hate the keto diet, I've personally worked with Olympians who perform at world-class levels, or have seen obese people lose over one hundred pounds and keep it off through the keto lifestyle. I'm not promoting keto, but I am promoting finding nutrition that works well for you, your lifestyle, and your doctor. Fuel your mind and body with quality nutrition. Nutrition is developmentally in the beginning stages, so expect to see even more research and findings to be released. New facts will arise, and I watch RDs and nutritionists argue about it all. They can't even agree. You'll basically find research to support and oppose practically anything, so don't entertain the madness. Do what's best for you. (And we'll discuss nutrition in greater detail in Part II.)

SUPPLEMENTS

I use supplements because our food doesn't have the quality it once did years ago. Working regularly with functional medicine doctors, they order a complete blood panel to see where I could use supplements to get to functioning and optimal levels. And with sports performance, I use the ones to give me the results I'm after, again, while working with my functional medicine doctor.

---

4   Dr. Corey said, "Over the years, we have come to find that ice is really only effective in the very acute stages of an injury to 'take the edge off' of the pain. Once we get out of that first twenty-four to forty-eight hours, you want to back away from the ice, as it is likely *slowing down* the healing process. The body has a very, very effective inflammatory process, which it needs to go through in order to heal something that is injured or irritated. It is very likely that ice slows down that response, which isn't a good thing—we *want* the body systems to go through that response to take care of the problem." So too much ice can slow down your body's natural response to heal. Well, then, can heat help? Dr. Corey said, "Maybe, but I'm not necessarily a fan of heating pads either. Are they going to hurt anything? Very unlikely. But is the heat generated internally by the movement of the muscles and movement of the fluids of the body a much better solution? Absolutely. Long story short, you need to *move*."

STRENGTH TRAINING

Every sport uses strength training to increase performance, strength, overall health, mental health, and better joints. I'll talk more about this in future chapters.

MINDFULNESS

The greatest athletes and minds around the world meditate. That should say enough. I've used *Five Good Minutes* by Jeffrey Brantley, MD, and Wendy Millstine, as well as the Headspace App.

PRAYER

The power of prayer is life changing. You can start with devotionals like *Jesus Calling, Sacred Romance,* or *The Purpose-Driven Life.* Keep a prayer journal and write out your prayers and see them answered. The most powerful thing in the world is belief.

QUALITY SLEEP

I must admit that until I started treating my sleep as something sacred, I wasn't recovering at the rate that I needed to. I knew the mindset of hustling hard and sleep was minimal. Sleep really is sacred and crucial to the mind and body, and it took me changing my mindset and priorities before treating it as something sacred. No, you won't sleep when you're dead, and you'll miss out by sacrificing your health.

COUNSELING AND COACHES

Don't ever be above counseling and coaching. Life is full of obstacles, and we need more people on our team encouraging us forward.

Counselors and coaches are there to keep us moving and getting unstuck. Sometimes we are stuck in the ways we learned as kids, like the way I was with my hustling mindset. If you want to go far in life, you need a good team, and there is no such thing as a good team without a good coach.

OTHER SELF-CARE OR RELAXING ACTIVITIES

Float pool, infrared sauna, swimming, yoga, hiking, paddle boarding, being in nature, being in a good book, laughing with good friends, connecting with people you love, community, travel, journaling, weekend getaways, museums, cooking class, and retreats.

Apply some prevention, performance, and recovery tactics from the pros. Allow this to be part of your growth mindset.

Most of us don't have access or the disposable income to have a 24/7 medical team keeping you at your best, to point out that your everted foot is causing a gait imbalance that is later going to cause knee or hip pain or the way you deal with stress is pointing you into an addiction that ultimately wrecks your life and marriage. There are so many different scenarios, but being preventative and serious about our performance and recovery is crucial to our success in order to become a higher performer.

You don't need to do all the things the professional athletes do on a daily basis, because that's their job. However, learning from their mindset, habits, and how they perform and recover is worthy enough to adopt practices from.

Your self-care and health should be a priority. It won't be cheap, and I pay for my functional medicine doctor in cash simply because I know that's how and where I'll get the best care and results for my health, and insurance doesn't cover that. If your wellness isn't a priority now, you'll spend more time on your illness later, and I'm sure you don't want that.

Mindset, however, is free. Self-care practices are great tools for your mind and body to recover and perform at a much healthier and sustainable rate. Steal some ideas and practices for yourself; I know I do.

If you are going to learn from somebody, it may as well be the pros!

MEASURE AND REEVALUATE FOR YOUR SUCCESS

I loved sitting with the medical team, coaching staff, physical therapists, athletic trainers, and high-performance director, discussing each player and their treatment needs. Sitting in chairs, facing the big-screen TV, playing videos of every player to see where their strengths, weaknesses, and imbalances were, a plan was created to correct and coach the player to greatness.

Without this plan and evaluation, they could be more prone to injury and wreck their season or career. An injury costs the team money and causes the player to lose value. It takes the entire medical team and staff to keep a player playing his best, not just a hardworking hustler ego.

As a business owner, you are measuring return on investments. As an athlete, you are measuring your goals, points, and assists. You make goals to continue growing, reevaluating, and to see where the problem could be to overcome or make you stronger.

There are always goals. Always something to strive for to beat who and what you were yesterday.

Part of seeing how far you can go needs to include a recurring evaluation where you can see where the imbalances are that can keep you from greater success. This is preventative and proactive thinking.

You don't wait until you have a heart attack to lose the weight. You don't wait until the affair to fix your marriage. You don't wait until the stroke to manage your stress. Be proactive and preventative.

When anything is out of balance, whether it's your hip, big toe, stress levels, nutrition, or relationships, it creates a weakness keeping you from reaching your full potential. Be willing to be the healthiest and fittest you have ever been. Be willing to be preventative and proactive.

TAKING MY OWN ADVICE

The year 2020 threw me for a loop, as I think it did for most of us. Whereas some got in the best shape of their lives and were winning fitness competitions, others were just trying to do their best and keep their head above water.

In 2020, I was the latter.

In case you were and still are struggling from the pandemic that started in 2020, you can still recover and get back to kicking ass, but you have to focus on the recovery first.

I went from cooking clean, high-protein recipes to wandering down the frozen foods section in Target, looking for the easiest premade meal I could find. I wanted something that I could just heat in the oven and call it a day. Like, let's just survive and keep this as simple as possible.

I didn't care if it was gluten-free, organic, full of protein, or healthy in the slightest bit. It was food on the table, and we were doing our best. Seriously, that was the best that I could do. And it was hard.

I think many people were just trying to do their best, and doing their best might be Stouffer's family-sized pot pie or takeout.

But why was 2020 so hard on me? Well, by the beginning of the pandemic, I was pregnant for the second time in a year. The first one we lost. The second one I went into labor and lost.

A couple of months later, I was forced to shut down my spa and somehow pay overhead, and my husband lost his job, too.

I had pretty much already finished writing my book, but with day-care closed, I was trying to edit it with my three-year-old at home. So that wasn't happening at all. Ha!

I took a leap of faith and hired a "business coach" who took $8,000 without fulfilling promises, and then I was pregnant with the third baby in a year. I was bedridden, hemorrhaging for months, and sleeping twenty-two hours a day.

It was a blessing in disguise my husband had lost his job because he kept our three-year-old alive when I could barely get out of bed.

Sadly, I went into labor, losing the third baby in just one year.

Because COVID-19 restrictions wanted to keep people out of the hospital as much as possible, I went through five manual D&Cs that summer. The pain was so intense that I almost passed out on the table. I could feel them ripping things out of me. Blood was everywhere, covering the doctor and ultrasound technician.

The procedure failed so many times, and it had to be repeated with each pregnancy. Finally, the fifth one was performed under anesthesia. Even then, my body still thought I was pregnant and continued to bleed for at least another month.

Each experience added more trauma.

It was so traumatic that somehow even though I am not pregnant, my body still responds to food as if I am. Most food makes me sick to even think of, so eating less of the wrong foods have actually made me gain weight. And then not being able to eat the right food to fuel me dramatically affects my workouts. Sadly, I couldn't even follow my own advice in this book to eat enough of the right foods, other than dialing back my intensity and expectation to focus on healing.

My husband and I have been doing our best by working through grief and loss, holding on to faith, being raw with God, and sometimes getting angry.

I'm sharing not for sympathy but to encourage, motivate, and inspire you that anyone can have those days, seasons, or years. But there comes a point where you are ready to get out of your funk and take the next step.

I have been getting better, but it took some creativity.

My husband and I have been walking with God through this. It hasn't been easy, but I couldn't imagine walking this out without Him.

I didn't need to just power through, hustle, and just get over it. We both needed to recover. Not just me but my husband watching me in agony as I was in labor too early, feeling helpless.

Our mindset, overall health, and self-care was and still is absolutely crucial to our performance.

I had to recover to get back out in the world and kick ass again. You may want to keep going, but recovery is just as important as training.

I couldn't work out like I wanted. I couldn't eat like I know I needed to. I almost had to have a blood transfusion, so lots of rest was most important. I focused on quality sleep, rest, physical therapy, chiropractors, working with a functional medicine doctor, and taking the right supplements. To work with my issue with food, I started ordering a food delivery service to ensure better nutrition.

Once I was ready to measure and reevaluate my success, I looked at my one-year-from-now goals and made sure the things I was doing aligned with getting me there. I've been working closely with functional medicine doctors, regularly getting blood work done, monitoring my thyroid, going to counseling as an individual and as a married couple, getting massages, chiropractic, physical therapy, being in nature, taking naps when I need to, saying no when it isn't a hell yes...not to mention lots and lots of prayer.

Now that you understand how to apply what the pros do to perform higher, Chapter 3 will show you how you can adjust your personal and professional dial for your own life and goals.

KEY TAKEAWAY

Wherever you are, you need rest. You need recovery. You need a healthy mindset, and you can't have that without healthy self-care practices.

Brendon Burchard also found that one common denominator of high performers is that they overcome loss better than others. So we need to deal with losses, because you can overcome.

Don't just keep hustling without a proper mindset and recovery to move on.

Without it, you won't be able to perform as well as you are truly capable of.

HIGH-PERFORMANCE EXERCISE

1. After reading different examples of what the pros do, what are new habits and self-care practices you would like to add to your life? Be sure to practice the mindset of professional athletes to make your self-care a priority.
2. Believe in yourself and your one-year-from-now exercise you did in Chapter 1. Your choices should help you move in that direction. Don't just read the exercises, but put them into practice daily.
3. Practice visualizing your life wheel goals and one year from now every morning before you start your day.

CHAPTER 3

—————

ADJUSTING YOUR DIAL FOR INTENSITY, LONGEVITY, AND PERFORMANCE

Before my first bodybuilding competition, I remember standing in line waiting to get my dark orange spray tan. It was my first time spray tanning, and I didn't know what to expect. It was late and all the competitors were exhausted.

While we all stood around, someone next to me asked, "Why are you here?"

I'm not a girl for small talk, so I liked her style to start off with something good. I looked down to think of a response and said, "Because it's the only thing I can do."

She seemed perplexed, although that wasn't my intent. I could simply answer that I was there for a spray tan, but that was too obvious. That's about as meaningless as talking about the weather.

"What do you mean?" she asked. "Most people won't ever attempt what you are about to do. How is this the only thing you can do?"

I explained that the previous year, I had gone on a snowboard tour and attempted racing professionals on thirty-plus-foot jumps.

After doing a few practice runs on the course, both of my feet were numb from my brand-new boots, so I untied them to walk around and get some circulation and feeling back into my toes. I intended to tie them when my name was announced to get into the start gate, but that very important detail left my mind.

The boots support ankles to give us snowboarders and skiers the ability to do crazy jumps. Since my boots were untied, I literally heard both ankles snap as I attempted to land after being about eighty feet in the air.

In the emergency room, doctors told me that both ankles were crushed, and the major weight-bearing joints of the ankle (the talus) were not only broken but had completely snapped in half and were displaced with multiple bone fragments.

As I was recovering from my injuries, I prayed on how to use my situation as a gift, and the only thing I could think of doing was a fitness competition. So I started training and dieting while rehabbing my ankles.

As I had lain on my parents' couch with casts on both legs up to my knees, having to army-crawl with my legs held off the ground behind me when I had to go to the bathroom, God shaped my perspective. He reminded me of stories in the Bible about the three men who received talents. One buried his, the second spent his, and the third invested and was able to give back more than what he was originally given. "God," I spoke out loud, "I want to be like the third guy."

I was in a difficult situation. I wouldn't be able to work for months. My home wasn't wheelchair accessible, and I just didn't know how I was going to afford to live and pay bills. But God showed me how to look at what seemed like an impossible situation and see it as a gift.

I didn't want to just heal and go back to the busy life I was living before. Nor did I want to pretend this event had never happened.

"I wanted to give God back more than what was given to me," I told the lady as we waited.

It's been just one way I choose to worship God.

My name was called to get tanned. When I went behind the drapes, I learned that I had to be completely naked, spreading arms and legs like a starfish while my body was painted a shade I'd never seen before. I later learned this ridiculous color was so that judges could see your lines and definition more clearly under powerful stage lights. A bad tan could cause you to be easily overlooked by the judges.

Friends sneaked in and held box fans aiming at my skin to be sure the orange-brown glow would be dried enough so I could finally go back to our hotel and sleep.

I finished in the top five the next day and began a hunger and curiosity to learn more about this sport and get even better.

I signed up for the Arnold Classic not even a year after both of my legs were still in casts, and I placed fifth among some of the most intimidating physiques from around the world.

I didn't just want to see how far I could go, but I wanted to learn as much as I could from the best from around the world.

That's when I introduced myself to John Meadows, International Federation of Bodybuilding (IFBB) Pro and world-famous bodybuilder and coach.

DISCOVERING MY DIAL

John Meadows and I worked out at the same gym. Apparently, he had seen me training while both of my legs were only partially weight-bearing and I had to use scooters and wheelchairs to move about. I carefully used my arms to lift my body from the scooter to sit on machines to train my upper body, and then I was restricted to swimming only or light resistance on recumbent bikes for my rehabbing ankles and legs.

Even though I had two shows under my belt, including one of the most intimidating ones from around the world, I wanted to understand more and do better. John took me under his wing and helped me find even greater transformation and success. I learned I was working ineffectively like the majority of competitors did, and he showed me how to not waste time in the gym.

He showed me how to train only three or four days a week with minimal cardio, while mostly everyone else focused on cardio almost every day, sometimes twice a day, plus lifting. So much unnecessary time.

Mostly because of John Meadows, I went on to win many more shows in the figure division and was ranked in the top twenty best physiques on bodybuilding.com, top ten nationally, and I nationally qualified multiple times again (in figure as well as in snowboarding since my injuries).

But I was exhausted. I was advancing as an athlete and as a business owner, but my health was wrecked.

Then I added a new baby to the mix. I started my new website and writing a book. And my health completely crashed.

I already knew I had hypothyroid Hashimoto's, which is slow metabolism, lethargy, and a cloudy mind that made me feel like I was sedated most of the day.

I was so tired that most days I felt like I needed to manually hold my eyelids open because they were so heavy. I could sleep for twelve hours and still feel like I could sleep more. I eventually got so tired of forcing myself through diets and training to finally get to the root of it.

After working with John, I knew how to lift weights and exactly what to eat to be strong and lean, despite how sluggish I felt.

My traditional doctor wanted to manage my thyroid and prescribed antidepression and anxiety medication. I am more into holistic health and getting to the root of things, so instead, I consulted functional medicine doctors. We did extensive blood, saliva, and urine tests. My traditional doctor saw the tests and said everything was fine. He said, "Your antibodies are high, but that's just because you have thyroid disease, and there isn't anything you can do about that."

Functional medicine looks at deeper levels to get to the root of what can be causing things. My functional medicine doctor said, "Well, no wonder you feel like shit."

He listed all my deficiencies and told me why my hormones, mind, and body were crashing. He showed me that my stress tests were through the roof and told me that I needed to make rest my focus and to stop lifting weights until we got my stress under control.

That was really extreme for me to not lift weights, but I understood if I wanted to have another baby and get my health optimal, what mattered was being as healthy as I could be for my situation. For me, that meant sleeping as much as possible, lowering my expectations, and fueling my body where I was deficient.

Ironically, I was in the middle of writing a course and an e-book on managing stress. I had to chuckle and I put it away and focused on managing my own stress. I wanted my mind and body to be as healthy as possible, so healing and rest became my new goal, not being ripped.

I learned that I needed to adjust my dial of how I approached my life. I'd had the intensity turned up way too high for too long.

Being able to have a different perspective on my life helped me look at all of this as a gift. I was able to adjust the dial at how intense I wanted to be, what my goals were going to be, and how to adjust along the way. I adjusted my own dial to focus on sleep, eating more, seeing functional medicine doctors to get optimal health again.

And you can learn how to use this dial for your own life, too.

ADJUSTING THE DIAL FOR YOUR OWN LIFE

Maybe you can relate to where I was before I discovered my dial. You want to get in shape, get lean, get strong, and look like you know what you are doing in the gym. You get your workout plan or hire a trainer and start your diet. You are serious about dropping weight and pretty intense about it; maybe you even say on a scale from zero to ten, you are at a ten for intensity.

But then work is backing up, the dog throws up, you step on your kids' Legos, and your projects are not being completed as planned. You are working extra hours, stressing out because you just need to get this one project done, but then you realize one project rolls into the next. Maybe you caught a cold. You are exhausted.

But instead of dialing slowly back from ten, you jump off the wagon completely, start ordering carryout, stressing about the stress, and you're back to putting the important things on the back burner—things like your health, your exercise, nutritious food, family, personal development, and your faith. The things that bring you joy are now in the distance, hoping you'll get to it again, whether that's yoga, hiking, or having a good cigar.

You abruptly drop from ten to zero.

Instead of being at a full-on ten or a dead-stop zero, I want you to learn that you can adjust your dial in different areas, moving up or down as needed to meet the stresses in life. And you can adjust that dial for intensity, longevity, and performance.

ADJUST YOUR DIAL OF INTENSITY

Nearly everyone wants good health. They want to feel good, look good naked, be confident, feel desired, and live a long and purposeful life. We aren't getting there when we are ignoring the need for our mind and body to be renewed and taking care of our overall health.

In whatever time you have been on this earth, you have probably realized there is no such thing as a pause button in life, not even during the year 2020. It just doesn't exist, but somehow we live our lives like we will be able to find that pause button.

Think about it, especially when it comes to diet and exercise, for example. How often do you decide you want to be strong and lean and then you do some fad diet or something to lose a bunch of weight and sweat like crazy at the gym every day until something happens? Then you stop completely, and you tell yourself you will start again next week or the week after that.

So here is where I teach you a trick to not only controlling your productivity and achieving more while doing less, but even how you can control your diet and exercise instead of jumping off the ship. Your health is crucial to getting to your future self and keeping those lasting changes!

Instead of starting again, starting over, and feeling frustrated, defeated, and like there's not enough time, you can adjust your dial of intensity.

Imagine your fitness like a dial that goes from one to ten.

If you dial it up to a ten, what would it look like?

- What would your workouts look like?

- What would your diet look like?
- What would your overall life look like?

If you dialed it down to a one, what would that look like?

- Then what would your workouts look like?
- What would your diet look like?
- What would your overall life look like?

Where is your dial set right now? Do you want to adjust it? Could you move it up just a notch?

Or maybe this is the crazy time where you usually jump off the ship and burn it, but instead, can you just turn down that dial so you are still in control and your ship is still moving forward?

It really isn't all or nothing. You really don't need to jump in as a ten, and then jump off when life gets hard. You have the power to adjust it down to nine, eight, seven, six...whatever you need.

And when you choose the number on the dial that is best for where you are right now, give 100 percent there. Being 100 percent at a four is completely different than being 100 percent at a ten, and it's completely okay to be okay with that. Give yourself that permission.

You have the power in your own hands. What makes the most sense to you right now, in this period of your life? What adjustment can you make? Does that dial need to go down? Go up a little? Stay the same?

Hopefully, you feel pretty good that you can control that darn thing. It's not an on-off switch, where it's either off or at a full-on sprint! You've got everything between one and ten to work with to keep you from jumping off your ship while also keeping the most important things in life the most important.

But maybe you do want to sprint in your life. And you can. There is a time and place. You can sprint, but you also need to figure in all your renewals to keep you, well...renewed.

You need to keep doing your life wheel of the ten areas every Sunday. And visualize your one-year-from-now and life wheel goals every single morning. Don't sprint while letting the other areas of your life fade away or forget the direction your ship is heading. You will kick ass at life holistically, not just obsessing about any one thing, and without compromising your well-being or relationships. This is what will bring you renewed and increasing joy!

I remember where I lived in the season after I crushed my ankles. The front door, like any front door, had a porch light. This one was different, though. Maybe it was a poor design or the cover of it flew off during a storm, but the light did not have a cover on it.

I gagged almost every time I was at my own front door because the porch light became a morgue for hundreds or thousands of moths. They were so obsessed about the light that they didn't realize they were flying into their certain death. Nothing else mattered.

That's what obsessing about just one thing can do to you, like any idol. Bring you to your own morgue and it's too late to realize anything else mattered.

Don't be that moth. There is more to you and your life than that.

ADJUST YOUR DIAL FOR LONGEVITY

Using the dial helps you adjust to where you are and where you want to go. By continuously jumping off the ship instead of adjusting your dial, you learn that when you decide to get back on the ship, you have to start all over, leading to feelings of defeat, failure, and shame.

But what if you didn't have to have defeat, failure, and shame as part of your dial?

Many live in this cycle that usually begins with a New Year's resolution. They typically jump on the ship thinking they need to eat and work out at the intensity of a ten until they meet their goal... or until something happens (stress, injury, sick kid, sick parent, family drama, etc.). Then they jump off the ship until they put out whatever fire is going on and go back to old habits.

They feel defeated. They feel like they failed at being healthy. They feel shame once again, until they put out their fires and jump back in weeks or months later to start over again.

Stop starting over and doing that to yourself. Do what your mind and body really needs, especially as a high performer.

You are in it for the long haul, not just an intense sprint. Although the dictionary may define longevity as number of years lived, instead view it as John did: It's a lifestyle.

LONGEVITY IS A LIFESTYLE

Just a few years after I met him, John ran a seminar for the Arnold Classic with Drs. Eric Serrano and Scott Stevenson. He called me up beforehand and said, "Hey, Bailey, I need you to be there."

I said, "You got it, boss. I'll be there."

A whole lot of muscly people gathered in the downtown Columbus conference room. Of course, we were all geeking out on training styles and nutrition, but John really lit up when he shared how he profoundly touched, changed, and inspired the entire fitness industry.

You see, he added a special section in the seminar about lifestyle and longevity and why it is so important.

John said, "Longevity is important because the people that don't understand this balance are gonna burn out or they are gonna lose all the important things to them. Their family, friends, and social connections."

He said you have to get this. Mentally, not just physically.

He shared that his most successful time in bodybuilding was when he was focusing more on his kids, because it put that much more joy in his heart. "When I have that joy in my heart, I feel better and I train better."

That joy is part of what kept him going.

Very few people could grasp time like John did. He mastered time with sets, rest, and recovery before his next training, meal timing... as well as time with friends, time with his wife, time with his boys, and time with faith.

Time that ultimately ran out, as he passed away in his sleep at the age of forty-nine, in the summer of 2021. Knowing that our time here is limited is why John emphasized working your tail off but always balancing the more important things like relationships and overall well-being.

We never know our next day or our last breath. Whether we will be ninety-nine or forty-nine. That's part of what he wanted you to get so bad. The longevity that he spoke of isn't just defined as how many years a life would live but about a meaningful, impactful, joyful, and present life.

ADJUST YOUR DIAL FOR PERFORMANCE

You are reading this book to learn how to be fit while being or becoming a higher performer. Part of doing so is learning your dial and how to adjust it so you are always keeping your health at the forefront.

Without optimal health, you simply won't be the higher performer that you have the potential to be, so let's speak into your potential and starve anything less than that. If you want to feed into the part of you that is "less than," then this book is not the right fit for you.

You have dreams and potential, and the only thing separating you is in your own mind. If you struggle with this, then go feed your faith.

You have already completed and set goals for the ten areas in your life wheel that help lead to performing higher overall. But when you pour your faith into those ten areas, there is no stopping you.

The most powerful tool in the entire world is not greed, money, or fame; it is the power of belief. Belief is what changes you from the inside out. Belief is what changes cultures and the world. Belief is something that can start so small and create lasting change, whether good or bad.

Think about it. There are extremists who truly believe murder is a good thing to do, so they do it in honor of their god. It doesn't make the belief right, but the belief is still strong enough to change them from the inside out ending the lives of others and themselves. Use the power of belief for good within you and your world.

If you begin believing in your potential and speaking into that and feeding that belief, all of your energy goes into it.

If you believe as much as you breathe, there is no stopping you. There would be no jumping off the ship. There would be no waiting for tomorrow or next year's resolution. There would be no more waiting until things are less stressful.

Start feeding into your faith, your belief, and your dreams, and starve out anything else that doesn't belong there.

Belief is the most powerful tool in the world and you have the key to unlock it. Nobody else but you.

What do you want to believe for as a higher performer? Do you want to be more successful in your craft or calling, while being more present in life, enjoying it, and being happily married? Do you want deep connections with your kids?

Stop and paint a picture in your mind of what you want to believe for. Write it down somewhere and make all your thoughts and actions move toward it. Focus on what matters most in life.

Do you see yourself growing old with someone? What does your marriage look like? How are you going to keep it strong and work out conflict? Are you going to jump off that ship too and start with a new one? What traits are you looking for in a spouse? What emotions do you want to feel? What grace are you willing to give? What will dates look like? How intimate will your conversations be? Or will you be so focused on your success that you become strangers in the same house?

What do family dinners and holidays look like? How important are they to you? Do you laugh together? Play games together? Or do you sit on couches and everyone is on their separate device? Are you going to kids' events? Part of their lives? Are you an example to your kids to how they will love and be loved by their future spouse someday?

What does your business and personal development look like? Are you complaining about the people at the top and only willing to do the minimal effort? Are you learning as much as you possibly can at whatever level you are now to become even more with it? Are you learning how to make yourself indispensable and valuable? Are you dreaming and bringing value? Are you ethical? Are you investing into your own growth? Are you in mastermind groups to expedite your growth and problem solving instead of re-creating the wheel?

What kind of people are you with? What kind of people do you want to be with? What kind of person do you want to become?

What does your health look like? Are you getting by without a plan but not feeling your best? Are you going to wait until you get a diagnosis before you make your health a priority? Are you at the gym?

Are you taking hikes? Are you treating symptoms but not getting to the root? Are you a runner? A lifter? Maybe for fun become a spin class instructor or snowboard instructor? How good do you feel? Do you have energy? Are you tired? Are you keeping up with your future grandkids? Are you managing your stress well? Are you making self-care more of a priority?

Visualize it all.

Visualize you and who you want to become and begin speaking life into it. Speak faith into it and begin believing for it.

How healthy do you want to be? What kind of joy do you want to have?

Think of the things you'd like to do and that would bring you joy. Then think of what capabilities you would need to get there.

YOUR DIAL IN ACTION

Let's see what it could look like when you adjust your dial instead of going full speed and then abandoning ship.

From zero to ten, how intense can you be with your training and nutrition right now?

I love training and eating at a ten. This means lifting weights three days a week, one to three days of high-intensity interval training (HIIT), nutrition supplements for best results and recovery, and dialing in my nutrition.

But not everyone starts at a ten. Maybe you start at a six, just getting to the gym, learning how to use the machines, how to use great form, and fueling your body with great nutrition. If you haven't lifted weights in a long time, maybe you start lifting about 60 percent of the weight that you think you can lift. This helps protect your joints.

As you get stronger, you can slowly increase that 60 percent to 65 percent and then 70 percent. Each workout allows you to feel yourself getting stronger and wanting to be challenged more, and you can increase the weight.

Then maybe you are learning how to eat better. So instead of eating an egg sandwich every morning from the drive-through, you opt for cooking breakfast at home and bringing a protein shake and a small handful of nuts to work as a mid-morning snack.

You start getting the hang of it, and it isn't as complicated as you thought it would be, so you turn up the dial to a seven. You are increasing the intensity at the gym all while staying safe. Instead of eating out for lunch, you bring a lean protein, carb, vegetables, and a small portion of fat (extra virgin olive oil or nut butter, for example) for your lunch.

Then maybe you have a trip or you just want to challenge yourself to see how much of a transformation you can make. So you increase your dial from a seven to a ten, which also means adding twenty to thirty minutes of HIIT cardio a couple of times a week after lifting. You start timing your meals for maximum results and get into supplements for performance and recovery.

But then life happens. We all have bad days. Stress comes for us all.

TELL YOUR STRESS WHERE TO GO

Who isn't busy? Who isn't stressed? Regardless of what level you are at, more than likely, you are stressed. Stresses are inevitable in life.

It's not about avoiding stress but about learning to respond better to it when it happens. With the dials, you have the power to respond better to the stresses, control your nutrition, training, and overall wellness in order to perform even higher.

Whether you are trying to simply provide for your family, learning to start your first business, how to expand it, how to invest, or how to manage thousands of employees, it all involves stress. It's up to you how you manage it, and don't wait until you're dead.

Instead of jumping off that ship and taking orders from that stress, you need to know that you are empowered to tell that stress what to do. You are empowered to adjust your dial. You don't look longingly at your schedule in hopes of living the life you dream of, and to be able to get to the gym again someday, and to start eating healthy again someday, but you take that stress by the horns and you tell it what to do.

Every time stress likes to show its face, I look at it and tell it where to go. Then I adjust my dial to be more proactive about it. Stress won't own me.

For example, something that brings me a lot of joy is snowboarding. Maybe I'm not trying to qualify for the Olympics anymore, but for fun I still compete and teach as a snowboard instructor. In the winter season, I know how much joy it brings me, so I intentionally dial back business deadlines and projects so I can play. If I try to maintain or increase stressful demands while also committing to a work schedule for our local ski resort, it's not exactly a wise choice.

You may be thinking, "Wouldn't it make sense to just not teach snowboarding?"

Perhaps it would. But I do it because I have the tendency to be a workaholic, so I have to be fierce when it comes to choosing play-time. Not to mention, play is also a way of managing stress.

In order to do it, I have to adjust the dial on my workload and budget my time.

When my husband and I first got married, we took Dave Ramsey's Financial Peace University, an eight-week course on finances. Dave said, "You budget so you can tell each dollar where to go instead of wondering where it went." You have the power to tell each dollar where to go.

You have the same power over your life and over your health.

You have the power to tell that stress where to go and how to manage it, or else it's going to manage you.

Being in the fitness industry for so long, it was extremely difficult to change my mindset and goals to put more focus on my health and healing rather than being stronger and maintaining my identity as a competitor.

But I wasn't the only one. There are many people who reach heights, and to not stay there is failure and taking on shame instead. Their identity was in how they looked, regardless of what was or wasn't on the inside.

Here, my traditional doctor was advising antidepressants, and my functional medicine doctor was showing me how my entire body was crashing and what I needed to do to heal and fix it.

I opted for healing it.

Sometimes taking a few steps back is what you need to heal and to have a clear perspective. Pushing your dial at a ten 24/7 is begging for a shutdown.

I gave myself permission to go to bed early and sleep until the baby woke up. Usually when she napped was when I crammed as much work as possible from home, such as emails, websites, posts, and building my courses. I had to get in my head to give myself permission to take a nap when she napped and to not let myself feel guilty about it. This wasn't for a few months; I did this for over a year. I learned that I really needed to guard my sleep instead of sacrificing it for work because if I did, I would be putting myself in danger, not only my health but as a high performer.

PERFORMING HIGHER WITH A LOWER DIAL

None of us get through life without hearing bad news.

I remember the day I received the text about my dad's diagnosis: "It's ALS."

I lived over two hours away and had to carefully manage my time for running a business, training, and planning a wedding. There were times I could still train and diet at a ten for the sake of my sport, but I stayed at a ten when I could have dialed it back.

I kept hustling hard, not willing to back down. I made a point to keep my dial at a ten for far too long and my health paid for it. I didn't realize I could adjust my dial instead of living at that ten through all the stresses I carried on my shoulders.

Thankfully, with amazing functional medicine doctors and testing, we were able to get my health back under control. Thankfully for me, it wasn't something more life threatening—but it could have been.

Be empowered to know you can adjust your dial instead of thinking you always need to be at a ten or jumping completely off the dial when life gets hard. It's okay to find what works best for you. It doesn't need to either be a zero or a ten. You have two through nine to play with, too!

After my dad died and I started seeing the functional medicine doctor, it was eye opening for me to realize how much my mind and body needed to adjust my ten back to a two. I continued to eat healthy, eliminated everything that apparently my body was sensitive to, and focused on rest, sleep, naps, and eating more. I focused on being okay to not be ripped like the pictures showed in muscle magazines. I reminded myself every day that my identity was not in my achievements and to love my body in every step of the journey.

I had to remind myself to love my body as I gained weight in pregnancy as the sickest pregnant lady ever, to slowly coming back after the emergency C-section and having my pooch of a belly. To love my body as it grew a human and was trying to get healthier to grow another one. To love my body when I wasn't trying to look like I was going to step on stage again. Finally, to love myself more and find my identity in someone a little deeper than just a body.

I began to love how soft and feminine I could be and how ripped I could be if I wanted. I loved my mind and the way it could perceive what mattered most. The way I didn't jump off the ship, but I gave myself permission to not hustle so hard all the time, to simply adjust the dial along the journey of life.

Because that's what life is: it's a journey. It's a journey with speed bumps and crashes. It's a journey with success and failures, mountaintops and valleys, seasons of awesome and seasons of sadness. We can't always control all of those outcomes, but we can control the dial. We can control our mindset, our perspective, our faith, and our response.

I wrote a letter to myself. If you like writing, give it a try. Give yourself permission to do it and be what you need and want.

Dear Self,

It's okay to replenish yourself. It's okay to rest. It's okay to say no. It's okay to have boundaries to protect all that is sacred of you and who you are becoming. It's needed to give yourself permission to do all of these things because you can't be anything without it.

With all the goals, challenges, deadlines, and demands, where do you fit YOU in? Will you continue to give and give and give yourself away until you bleed and there is nothing left? Will you finally stop to see you need to be well and loved, too?

Continue to ignore it and it will continue to run you so dry that nothing will be left. Nothing will be able to pour out of you anymore. You'll run dry. You'll run depleted. You'll run until you can't run, but that's why this cycle must break.

It's time to choose self-love.

The cycle must break before you do.

If you want to have something to give, something to pass on, or someone to be or become, then you must do these things. Break the cycle before it breaks you.

You must. You can't put that off anymore. Your health depends on it. Your sanity depends on it. Your joy depends on it.

It's not about achieving anymore. It's about loving yourself a little bit more today than you did yesterday.

So go ahead and love yourself like the love you give everyone else, but this time, don't wait until there is nothing left. Light a candle, meditate, perhaps do nothing. Feel all the good feels of your most treasured memories. Know your worth and don't give it away for free. Sleep hard, get massages, and stop rushing. Keep only the kindest of friends, break off those that drain you. Speak life, love life, and live life.

You are a life worth loving, but you must be the first to show it.

Love,

Me

High-performance life isn't a sprint or a hustle; it's a dial. Part of performing even higher for a sustainable amount of time is learning how to generate your own energy without being burned out and exhausted, and being able to pour your energy into the areas that matter most—the ten areas in the life wheel.

So how do we generate more energy to keep this up? I'm so glad you are wondering this because I have it all laid out for you in Chapter 4.

KEY TAKEAWAY

To perform higher, learn how to adjust your dial, not press pause. Sprint hard when you can sprint, but ultimately you have a dial you can control to keep yourself on course.

There are no pause buttons in life. There is adapting. There is adjusting the dial. There is learning how to better manage your stress and generating even more energy to achieve more in less time. You can renew your mind to be even more productive and successful in every area of your life, and your workouts shouldn't be taking all of that focus.

HIGH-PERFORMANCE EXERCISE

1. You are in control of your dial through the ebbs and flows of life. Where are you right now in training, nutrition, and overall well-being?
2. What fitness and nutrition levels are best for you right now while keeping your relationships and overall well-being a priority?
3. Watch *Mary Poppins*, then *Saving Mr. Banks* as a date night or family night. (Note: *Saving Mr. Banks* is more for adults.) We'll talk about these movies again later in the book.

CHAPTER 4

—————

GENERATING YOUR ENERGY TO BE FIT AND A HIGHER PERFORMER

I had a first-time client come in for a massage. Jeffrey was extremely stressed out, bound up, had an intense personality, and he wanted me to fix everything.

The massage did not go very well at all. Jeffrey seemed to want to have control over every moment and would not allow his mind to relax. He said he wanted deep tissue, but he was so stressed and intense he propped his body up on the table and wasn't able to take a moment to relax.

I tried guiding him to relax mentally so his body would follow, but he didn't realize the connection between his mind and body. His controlling mind inhibited his body from relaxing, too.

The massage turned into life coaching and guided meditation in hopes to unlock his mind that was a tangled and stressed-out mess.

Jeffrey was a high achiever but only in one area, just like all the separate camps in the *Divergent* movie series. It was this extreme that brought him so out of balance that it greatly affected his life, body, and mind. If only he would see how much more he could achieve and grow if he wasn't so obsessed with one area and realize he could become a divergent, or an overall high performer.

As I attempted to give him the deep tissue massage he wanted, Jeffrey continued to hold his head and limbs off the table, while still trying to convince himself that he was relaxed. It was quite difficult to give him my trademark deeper work while his limbs were suspended in the air like a turtle lying on its back.

"Imagine your arm is like gelatin, and allow it to fall to the table," I told him in as soothing a tone as possible. "If you hold it up, you aren't exactly relaxing, ya know."

We had a lot of work to do. He wanted some serious deep work, but he wasn't ready. It's like the winters I teach snowboarding lessons and a bunch of kids want to do 360s off jumps, yet they can barely get off the chairlift or make it down the mountain without crashing. There are progressions that are important and necessary for a reason. Jeffrey learning how to let go and relax was one of them.

I was hoping that by the time he flipped over and his face was smashed down in the headrest looking at the ground, maybe he would start to shut his mind off instead of ordering me around and ruining his massage session.

While facedown, it is harder to lift your limbs off the table, but he still found a way. He said he wanted more pressure, all while every muscle in his body was contracted and tensed. It was difficult giving more pressure when he wasn't cooperating at all.

Jeffrey taking on more pressure wasn't the answer even though it's what he thought he needed.

That's when I had my revelation and felt God speaking to me about my own life. Just as the client thought he needed to take on more when he clearly couldn't, I was trying to take on more responsibilities when God said I shouldn't.

I almost stopped in mid-stroke down Jeffrey's unrelaxed back.

This entire fight on the massage table wasn't for my client at all; it was for me.

"It's not about how much you can take on, but how much you can let go" was what I heard in my spirit.

Just as I was attempting to coach this guy to let go, he just wanted to take on more, and he wasn't built or ready for it. In our minds, we think we can and should take on more, when clearly there are some things to let go of first.

I was doing all the things to take on more pressure in my own life, and that was weighing me down. I needed to live what I was teaching and coaching others to do.

GENERATING MORE BY DOING LESS

As Brené Brown said, "It takes courage to rest and play in a world where exhaustion is a status symbol."

People brag about being the busiest like it's a status symbol—to the point of damaging their health, life, faith, and family. If they don't brag, it's what they find their identity or self-worth in, when busyness can actually be the very thing that deflates what you are truly capable of. Doing more, achieving more, taking on more, and adding more busyness to your life isn't what matters most.

The answer isn't always more; in fact, most of the time, it's less. We can't pick up more if our hands are full. We can't take more pressure if we haven't learned how to manage the pressure we already have. If you want more, you need to learn to live with less and do what matters most first.

If not, you'll burn out. You'll get crushed. If you want to sustain High Performance and success for a long period of time while maintaining or improving your well-being and relationships, then you need to learn to let go and do less (just as John talked about at the Arnold Classic seminar I mentioned earlier). Do what matters most. Do what is essential. Learn boundaries to what you say yes to.

When you do this, you create space for your mind and body to achieve more, even while teaching yourself that it's okay to do less sometimes. You increase your productivity more than ever.

To get to the top and stay at the top, you'll need to generate and renew your own energy even when mentally, emotionally, or physically drained. Be religious about renewal practices for higher performance in the gym, business, and life.

Are you doing the things to become a vibrant leader, parent, business owner, employee, and athlete? Whatever you are, are you doing it with vibrancy, full of energy?

Be willing to put in the effort to be vibrant, to do the work to create that energy; it isn't as hard as you think. But you just can't expect it, wish for it, hope for it; you have to grab the bull by the horns and be willing to do what is necessary to have that kind of energy and become vibrant.

When you dream about the life you want, have you created the energy it will take to get it and keep it?

I'm not big on calculating calories or macros, but I am big on measuring the vibrancy of your mental, emotional, physical, and spiritual energy.

Make your mental, emotional, physical, and spiritual energy a very important part of your life. Not by energy drinks and another cup of coffee but by cultivating it through your raw self. Be honest with yourself about your energy levels, because your body could be telling you something. Without honesty, you could potentially miss the real reason why you lack the energy.

Energy is required for living. If you are living off fumes, then you are taking away from your own life, not making it any better. To be a high performer, you must be religious about this. If you want to kick ass at life, you need energy to maintain your well-being and positive relationships. That is something to take quite seriously. It's more important than obsessing about counting your macros.

That's why this book is so important. You really can have it all and be healthier, stronger, and leaner. But you can't do it while considering relationships and well-being to be less important. If you want to change the world and be the absolute highest performer that you can be, it starts within your heart and mind. From there, it shows in your family. What you do within your family, work, and all the people you meet is what matters most and changes the world—just like I learned from John and my own dad.

Working yourself into exhaustion and frustration does the absolute opposite. It damages your focus, your energy, marriage, family, and the hopes of leaving your best legacy.

It is your responsibility to create energy for your health, for your business, for your family, and for this world.

Think of the professional athletes as an example. They perform at that level because they take their energy and vibrancy seriously. It's just as important as the training itself. What good is an athlete who is driven into the ground without time to heal, ice, stretch, and rest well?

Think of yourself as that professional athlete. And your game is your high-performance life. If you want to perform higher, make greater income, make a bigger impact, have deeper relationships, a more fulfilling marriage, and amazing relationships with your kids, then you need to play like it and protect your energy.

If you are like me, you aren't lazy. In fact, you are the opposite. You want to do everything and want to do it well, but it's easy to get overwhelmed, and then you have to find the energy to keep going.

If you've read this far already, then that tells me you know this transformation won't happen magically. The magic happens by the action and belief you put in. It happens by creating the energy you need and wish you had.

But you don't have more time, so how do you create more energy?

So glad you asked.

It's not only by what you are willing to do but by also what you won't do. Things you say no to. Things on your not-to-do list. Even to the point of scheduling time for nothing.

SCHEDULE NOTHING AND YOU'LL BE MORE PRODUCTIVE

The CEO of LinkedIn intentionally scheduled thirty-minute slots in his calendar just to do nothing. Although some people thought this was crazy, it ended up creating more space in his mind and therefore much more productivity for his company.

Einstein said, "I think ninety-nine times and find nothing. I stop thinking, swim in silence, and the truth comes to me." We can learn a lot from Einstein and the LinkedIn CEO.

We cannot continue to pile up more and more on our shoulders and expect to perform well. We need to learn to perform better overall, and sometimes that means giving yourself permission to say no, to schedule nothing, to create space, and discover how much more productive you could be. The answer isn't always more; oftentimes it's less.

Just like this terrible massage session where the client just wanted to take more and more pressure but couldn't handle any of it. He needed to learn how to let go, not to flex his muscles and demand more. That way of life won't end well, and neither will the massage.

There are reasons for giving your mind permission to do nothing and rest: to be more productive, create more clarity, and generate more energy. Allowing time to rest and do nothing can play a strategic part of your recovery, renewal, and performance.

Without those three things, you won't be able to perform higher for a long period of time, and therefore you won't be the high performer you have the potential to be.

Oftentimes as part of a massage session, I include guided meditation or prayer in the beginning. Most people lie down on the massage table but are mentally still at work thinking about everything they need to do.

Part of serving my clients is to guide them to be mentally and physically present. We focus on their breath, the coolness of the air as they breathe it in through their nose, the weight of their bodies on the table, the warmth of the sheets, the sound of the music. We focus on bringing their shoulders away from their ears, all before the massage starts. Where the mind is, the body follows.

It's crucial to guide someone to leave work, to-do lists, and stress behind so that their mind and body can be renewed. It's part of allowing space for your mind to do nothing in order to rest and therefore become more productive.

It's a way to recharge your battery.

RECHARGE YOUR BATTERY ON A REGULAR BASIS

When you dream about the life that you want, have you created the energy it will take to get it and keep it?

Brendon Burchard talks about journaling every morning to

measure your energy. You can measure it physically, mentally, emotionally, and spiritually. You can make yourself more aware of it and be more intentional about creating space that allows your energy to increase.

By measuring your energy on a regular basis, you will become more in tune with when your battery is getting depleted and needs to be recharged.

You can also measure your vibrancy. How vibrant are you physically, mentally, emotionally, and spiritually on a scale from one to ten?

Stop and evaluate where you are so you can be vibrant in your life...not drained. It's important to adjust as needed to increase your vibrancy. That's part of generating and increasing energy along your journey.

What are you going to do to increase your vibrancy? Here are some ideas you can try.

EMOTIONAL IDEAS

- Cut relationship ties where needed
- Work with counselors who help
- Prayer and meditation
- Life-giving conversations

MENTAL IDEAS

- Books and podcasts that you enjoy
- Doing what it takes to find alone time to refuel your mind even if it's only five minutes

- Manage stress
- Not engaging in conversations (whether in person, in your head, or on social media) you don't need to be a part of
- Work with coaches and counselors

SPIRITUAL IDEAS

- Pray
- Worship
- Draw closer to God
- Prayer partner
- Tithe and give
- Devotionals

PHYSICAL IDEAS

- Activities you enjoy
- Optimal nutrition
- Massage
- Exercise
- Deep breathing
- Get better sleep
- Infrared sauna

If you are honest with yourself, where are you scoring? Choose one thing in each area that you can do that will increase your energy and vibrancy to keep you going strong.

WHEN YOU DON'T HAVE ENOUGH TIME

You may be reading this and thinking, "That's great, but I don't have enough time to be recharging my battery and regenerating energy."

I have news for you: nobody has enough time; that's why you need to be intentional with what you do with it. Prioritize what's important and start now.

It's important to create habits for a better well-being now so you don't have to pay for the damage later.

You must make the time. Create lists of what matters most and list priorities. One of my favorite lists is the "not-to-do" list. It's easy to pick up tasks that are distracting and stealing time. List them out and make a promise to yourself that you will do less of them, with the goal of doing none at all.

It's up to you to be the guardian of your time; it is sacred. Remember, out of seventy-eight years on this earth, only nine are yours.

With small amounts of time each day, you can create habits to build the lifestyle and mindset that you want. If you don't nurture those habits, then you are choosing to not build the higher performer you are capable of becoming.

In case you couldn't tell, I loved the *Divergent* movies. The main character didn't just classify in one area of expertise, but she was an expert in all areas, making her a divergent. What made a divergent so gifted was the fact that they could be so advanced and high performing in all areas, versus just one, like average people.

And that's what high performers are: divergents. They advance and perform high in all areas, not just one. And a little spoiler: even average people can implement habits each day to become a high performer, not just the divergents.

Learning renewal rhythms to generate more energy is one crucial step to doing so.

RENEWAL RHYTHMS TO GENERATE MORE ENERGY, FOCUS, AND INCOME

Okay, I have to tell you what a big deal this next lesson is. Multiple people paid $60,000 to learn what I am about to give you for the cost of this book.

Sometimes we take the free stuff for granted. When you get something for free, your eyes glance over it. When there is no skin in the game or value set into something, it doesn't create near as much importance to you. For example, if you paid $60,000 for coaching and retreats to learn something, you probably would be at the edge of your seat absorbing every moment. But if you got it for free, it wouldn't mean nearly as much.

So take this as seriously as you would if you'd paid $60,000 for it. Think of it as an investment in yourself, your future, your career, your personal development, and your goals—even though you paid much less for this book.

Okay, now are you ready to learn what a renewal rhythm is?

This renewal rhythm is a tool used by Burchard, other coaches, and high performers. It consists of having something you will look forward to to renew your mind and body every year, quarter, month, week, and day.

That's it.

Are you asking, "People paid $60,000 for that?"

Well, yes. When people realize how much more powerful and productive they can become when they renew their mind and body and invest into themselves, they get back more than just what they put in; that's why it's called an investment.

When you renew your mind and body, you are creating space in your mind to think clearly and creatively. You can come up with ideas that can save you a ton of money at work or make a ton of money, too. You can save your marriage. You can be more engaging, more present, and more productive. And the physical aspect? You aren't worried about your health, stress, anxiety, or blood pressure because you have been making your life wheel your priority.

You are happier, more joyful, healthier, more fit, and you benefit your company even greater. You take bigger steps toward your own goals and dreams.

Let's look deeper at the renewal rhythms to really get those benefits.

Think of taking a vacation every year. It can be big; it can be small; it doesn't matter. It just needs to be something you can look forward to and unplug, time off, to renew your mind and body. Whether you travel the world, go on some wild adventure, or keep it simple and go on a retreat with hikes and yoga. What matters is that it's something you unplug and invest into yourself and renew your mind and body.

Then you do something like this every quarter, every month, every week, and every day. Maybe you can't go on a tropical retreat every single day, but I'll break it down so you can have bite-size chunks.

QUARTERLY

Have something every quarter to look forward to. You can even use this as a way to reward the progress of your ship. Reward your joy that you have been working on, and amp up that joy even more by doing something every quarter. Again, it can be as big or small as you want. Something that has always sounded peaceful to me and I'll be doing soon is doing a silent retreat for a weekend in a monastery. Maybe you can do something for each season like hike, snowboard, kayak, or camp. Maybe it's a spa day. Maybe a yoga retreat or workshop, wine tasting, or an overnight stay at a cabin in the woods. Make a list of smaller things you could do every quarter that would be worth the return on investment for your mind and body that ultimately moves your ship forward because of that renewal.

MONTHLY

What recharges your mind on a monthly basis? Maybe it's giving time like serving in a homeless shelter or doing something outdoors. Maybe a drive to a favorite lake. Is there a place around you that you love to visit that recharges you? Or maybe it's hiring a sitter and locking your bathroom door, lighting candles, playing music, and soaking in an Epsom salt bath with a glass of wine. Something I'm inspired by is one of my best friends who has been married for fifty years has had prayer groups for their married friends every month for as long as they've all been married. Yes, I want that. I find that renewing and refreshing.

WEEKLY

This one is a no-brainer for me. I love to worship in church. I'll have my prayer journal and write as I feel the Holy Spirit lead me. I might sit while everyone else is standing, just so I can write down the inspiration before I forget; I don't care. This renews my mind and spirit and calms my mind and body like nothing else. Think of something you can do weekly.

DAILY

Find something smaller and less intimidating to look forward to daily.

The highest performers around the world meditate twice a day. If this is new to you, don't make it complicated. You can close your eyes and listen to guided meditation on YouTube or on a free app to get started. Or just visualizing and feeling the feels of your one-year-from-now or your life wheel goals. Close your eyes, go there, and feel it before you get out of bed every single day. Meditate and feel the feels of what it would be like to be where you want to be in every area of your life. To be at your healthiest, strongest, and happiest. Meditate on what you wrote for previous chapters. Print it out and use it as screen saver.

Think how you want to feel physically. I like being strong and lean, so I focus on lifting weights and having a high-protein diet. I'm also concerned about my immunity level to fight off sickness and infections, so I eat quality food, not just because it fits in my macros, and I increase cardio training for overall metabolic health. I keep it simple as to what I'm teaching here so I can live the life I love, too.

You need something small, even on a daily basis to renew your mind and body. Maybe you can't be on vacation every single day of your life, but you niche it down to where you can find things that will renew your mind and body every day, every week, every month, every quarter, and every year.

Sure, you can hustle between those times, but renewal needs to be part of that to keep your ship running and powered up. It's how the professional athletes stay on top of their game by including recovery and renewal as part of their performance plan.

Write down ideas for daily, weekly, monthly, quarterly, and yearly renewal goals. This is part of recharging and powering up your ship full speed ahead. This, my friend, is what many people paid $60,000 for, and you got it for free.

Take this and apply it, as if you had paid $60,000 for it, please. You'll see and feel the results for yourself.

THE $60,000 TOOL

Renewal is crucial to your mind, body, success, income, well-being, health, relationships . . . ALL OF IT! You are losing out on so much more without guarding this simple tool. Decide the ways you can renew yourself on a regular basis to increase your overall success.

Yearly Renewal: Date _____

This can be a big vacation where you unplug, go on an adventure, and be completely renewed. Retreats, world travel, beach vacation, mountain vacation. What renews you?

Quarterly Renewal, Every Season

Continue to enrich and renew your mind and body for dynamic and powerful quality outputs in the other areas of your life. Smaller version of your annual, i.e., yoga workshops, weekend retreats, wine tasting, ski trip in the mountains, beach vacation, etc. Include a deadline for each season or quarter.

Monthly Renewal

Choose what works best for your schedule to complete by the end of every month. This could just be a visit to a healing or rejuvenating place that is special to you, or visit somewhere new. Do what renews you on a monthly basis (hiking; road trips; weekend getaways; workshops for health, business, or marriage; etc.).

Weekly Renewal

Include your Life Wheel reevaluation as part of this (worship, church, small group meeting, yoga, be in nature, massage, chiropractor, other forms of self-care and treatment).

Daily Renewal

Morning routine, reading, meditation, and prayer. Visualizing and feeling the feels of your One Year from Now and Life Wheel.

JUST RELAX

Greg is a client I see every week. He's a successful entrepreneur who is married and has kids. He is also a high performer, as he seeks to do well in every area of his life, including keeping his well-being and relationships on the forefront.

I asked Greg if I could share his story in my book, and he kindly agreed to tell it. Here is Greg's story in his own words:

> I do not have a typical nine-to-five job; I work in several unrelated fields and consult, which has its pros and cons. I enjoy never being bored, but at times it can be demanding and stressful. On the upside, I get the flexibility to do the things that are most important to me.
>
> Unfortunately at certain points in time, I have not had enough flexibility and something has to suffer. I let my physical and sometimes mental health pay the price.
>
> When I first started to really invest in my health, I was burning out mentally and had also recently suffered a serious physical injury. Over time, the deep tissue therapy has done wonders for my mind and body, but initially it was not that easy to get into. It can be painful!
>
> But working with Bailey, I was able to learn to almost get into a meditative state and learn to breathe through it all. Although breathing is something we all do every day, it is different when it comes to completely relaxing. I was able to learn to completely relax my muscles so that my body could heal but also relax my mind and think of absolutely nothing, which was a much-needed break in my hectic schedule. Being able to truly think of nothing was quite a challenge for me. Even while working on one project, I am thinking of what I need to do on another project.

Once I was able to relax, I was also able to get back into working out, perhaps not at my peak, but at a level that was helping improve my overall health and well-being. It also reenergized my mind so I could think clearly and attack the problems I had to deal with that week more effectively and efficiently.

Due to things that happen in life sometimes, I am not always able to stick to the therapy schedule I have created for myself. For example, during the pandemic lockdowns, I noticed my physical and mental performance began to slip over time, as I was letting old habits creep back into my life and no longer taking the time to actually look after myself.

That's when I realized the value of the work that Bailey was teaching me to do. Some of it seems so basic and obvious, but most of us really don't spend enough time on our body and minds, especially if there is an important work deadline involved.

KEY TAKEAWAY

Take a much-needed break in your hectic schedule. Cherish it like it's $60,000, maybe a little more. That investment into your very being (physically, mentally, emotionally, and spiritually) can have a much greater return.

Imagine being strong AF in every area of your life, becoming that higher performer. You aren't just fit; you are more than that and then some!

HIGH-PERFORMANCE EXERCISE

1. "It's not about how much you can take on but how much you can let go."
   What should you let go of? What are some things to put on your not-to-do
   list that can be a distraction from where you need to go?
2. Rate your energy mentally, emotionally, spiritually, and physically from one
   to ten. What are some things you can do to feed each one to contribute to
   your vibrancy?
3. Plan in advance, and use this as a guide to generate more energy and increase
   your vibrancy. What will you do yearly, quarterly, monthly, weekly, and daily?

PART II

NUTRITION

I wanted to continue on my journey of healing my body of the lethargy from hypothyroid and get a little leaner at the same time, so I reached out to a registered dietitian. I explained that I was a busy business owner, a new mom, and trying to heal through better nutrition. I had a lot on my plate, so to maximize my time as a business owner, mom, and wife, I hired a professional to take care of the nutrition aspect for me so I could focus on the more important things.

Her response was macros.

I asked her, "Could there be certain foods I should be avoiding because of my thyroid? I noticed I feel really sluggish if I have more carbs and I'm not sure why. Could you help?"

She directed me to eat the highest amount of carbs I've ever eaten in my life, and my health worsened.

"Do you have a suggestion of meal plans or foods I should eat or should not eat so I can focus on feeling better while losing a little body fat?" I asked.

"You can eat whatever you want, just make sure it fits within your macros. You can eat the same thing every day if you want, or you can calculate each day as you go. It's up to you."

I was disappointed to receive this unhelpful response.

She was absolutely clueless about the nutritional help I had hired her for, but I continued to listen even though she seemed to have no interest in helping my gut heal.

It was a disaster.

Many high performers do this, and sometimes it's just a big disaster. They hire the trainers and nutritionists to save time so they can show up to the gym and have someone just telling them what to do. The trainers and nutritionists or RDs do the work, but remember to hire what you are looking for.

Just like any career, you'll have plenty of professionals and employees who just show up and do the minimum. Just because they have the certifications and alphabet soup behind their name, does not mean they can get you from point A to point B like you hired them to.

Take my initial career as another example. For more than twenty years, I have been doing private massage therapy sessions, and I've learned from my clients how most other therapists are. They've told me how they've gotten massages all over the world where it feels like they are just smearing lotion on them or just waiting for the time to pass.

You may have gotten a massage before and it wasn't that great of an experience, so you don't care to have that as part of your renewal or self-care routine. But in all honesty, you just had a bad massage and good therapists are rare to find.

It's the same thing with physical therapists. I worked in sports medicine as a teenager while in college, and not all therapists are created equal. It was just as obvious then; you could tell which ones took their job more seriously to get more results with their patients.

The same is true with hair stylists, doctors, virtual assistants, web designers, trainers, dietitians, and so on. If you want the best service and the best results, it takes going to the ones you know who can get them.

Someone once asked me why would they read my book if they could just hire a trainer or a nutritionist to do it for them. The quick answer is this: Not all trainers and nutritionists are created equal. Any trainer can get you to work out, can get you to sweat, can get you to show up, can get you to increase your heart rate. But none of that means you will get the maximum results that you want.

Just like nutritionists. You can hire a nutritionist just like I did because that's what they are trained to do, but it caused more harm than good for me. There is a reason you are still in the same place and with the same frustrations, and it's because you didn't know any better.

It's not your fault.

You did what you thought you needed to do, but you were led in the wrong direction. How frustrating is it to work as hard as you have been working and hardly see or feel any results?

You've been sweating, working out hard, showing up at the gym, listening to your trainer, restricting your foods but only seeing slow (if any) progress.

Most trainers at gyms have minimal experience, get a simple certificate online, and have a stamp to declare they can get you results, but there is more to it than that. You put your trust in them, that they could answer your problems, get you results, and finally feel better.

But instead, you are working harder than ever, and it seems impossible to reach your goal, let alone to stay there.

You need a more efficient plan where you get the results in less time, and you get to eat more food to fuel it all without it taking over your life. You can't be running on empty or poor fuel and expect a great finish.

Seasoned trainers are usually not personally training at commercial gyms, but that's where they get started. If you want results, you don't go where people are just getting started; you go where results are being made. However, it can be a good starting point. Starting somewhere is better than nothing, but when you want to get maximum results, it takes a different mindset.

Isn't it frustrating, though? It's frustrating to be trying your hardest every day but not seeing or feeling the results. Instead of feeling like you are making progress, you feel defeated. You feel depressed. You ask yourself why even bother and why try.

And then you think you have to be in the gym longer, diet harder, sweat more; becoming more and more obsessed while the rest of your life falls apart.

This is where the high-performance life comes in.

You really can excel in your fitness and nutrition while improving the other areas of your life. You really can make the improvements in all areas of life. You don't need to be stuck where you are. I mean, if you really want to stay there, you can, but something tells me you don't want to be if you are reading this book.

You can find a more sustainable method to be able to perform higher in all areas so you can have that overall lifestyle that you want and can have. It just takes a little adjusting of your dial.

CHAPTER 5

HOW TO GET EXTREME RESULTS IN MINIMAL TIME

"Excuse me, wow, you have a great butt!"

This is a sincere compliment that I've given others, and I haven't gotten punched in the face for it yet.

Thankfully, I say it in a noncreepy kind of way that makes people blush, yet you can tell they are happy that someone notices their hard work.

I know I love getting compliments.

Who doesn't?

The world could use a few more compliments, so I am always ready to dish them out. I can appreciate great sculpted eyebrows or a perky butt, but even more important are character traits. I may start with the brow and the butt, but I like getting to the stuff that really matters.

But to get that fine asset to make me want to stop a complete stranger, they aren't getting it by hanging out on cardio machines. They are not doing endless cardio and eating diet food.

Nope, those people get those chiseling eye-stopping physiques by lifting weights and focusing on nutrition.

THE BEST PHYSIQUES IN LESS TIME

Do you ever see people with strong and sculpted physiques, who have tons of energy and focus, and wonder how they do it?

Most of us want that type of physique.

I can't tell you how many times people have come up to me, excited to try giving up meat or to start jogging on a treadmill, thinking they'd make great changes. However, they soon give up because that's not how you see the results they were after. They are quickly disappointed and lose motivation.

Be honest with yourself. When you tell yourself you want to lose weight or lean down a little bit, you start eating salads and just aim to burn a lot of calories typically on a treadmill, right? Although a salad and a good run could be good for your health, it's not the magic pill to losing body fat and getting the most extreme results you are capable of.

If you want the fastest and extreme results in minimal time, it takes more than just eating salad, skipping breakfast, and being a hamster on a treadmill. Just as it takes intentionality to have a successful business, marriage, and team, it takes just as much intentionality in the gym, but this is how you do it in only three hours per week.

> High performers are efficient with time. They don't waste it.
>
> Don't waste time in the gym either.

You have a ton on your plate, and it's easy to spin out of control and not know where to start. You are balancing your business, new projects, dealing with urgent matters, making sure your wife feels loved, your kids feel engaged, and your dog gets walked. It can be overwhelming. So the last thing we need to do is make it even more overwhelming.

Hey, you've gotten this far. You can keep going. It's part of evolving, growing, and being challenged.

The trick is learning how to keep going without losing your mind, marriage, family, or business.

Let's not wait until shit hits the fan, things spin out of control, served divorce papers, or you get the diagnosis that finally makes you want to change. You aren't waiting for things to slow down, but instead you take responsibility over your own life.

You are reading this book because you are ready to make changes and healthier habits now and to become a higher performer, not just with your body but with your entire life. You already know that you can get any workout, diet plan, macros, or healthy recipes off the internet for free, but this one's different.

You are a high performer (or becoming one), so you need to think, live, eat, rest, and train like one. Part of being a high performer is having a growth mindset, not a fixed mindset where you limit your own potential. You can generate your own reality in your mind and make the changes needed to get the results you are after. If you want a successful career, marriage, family, and health, you must be an essentialist with your time management.

What will it take to shift from "salads and treadmill" thinking to maximum growth in minimal time? What will it take to stop fad diets and make that lifestyle change where you don't feel like you are a yo-yo anymore?

You are a max-results-type person in every area of your life. You want the most out of life and the God-given opportunities, and this is one of them.

There is more to being a high performer than counting every calorie you put in your mouth and being so focused on your body that you lose track of the quality of your entire life. If you want to perform higher and go to the next level, then you want more time to do what you want with your life and results to show, wow, and prove yourself.

In Part I, we dived into mindset to create lasting change. Now in Parts II and III, you can use the same mindset for your body and the results you want. First, you examine your nutrition, and then you learn my three-day-a-week weightlifting plan. You already wrote down what you want for yourself and what you want to feel. This is the plan to take you there. This is how you turn that dial up to a ten, to get extreme results in minimal time while living a high-performance life simultaneously.

If you want to jump in full throttle, this is the chapter for you.

HOW TO GET MAX RESULTS

Let's get straight to the good part where I tell you exactly how to get in the best shape of your life in the least amount of time so you can still focus on the important things in life: performing higher and being happier and more present.

If you don't want maximum results, that's okay because you can adjust your dial to your own intensity. If it's not a season to be a ten, then dial it back. Don't make it complicated.

I'm going to start off by showing you how to be at a ten with your training and nutrition to get the body and health that you want. The great part is that you can do it in only three to four days a week so you aren't neglecting marriage, family, goals, and all the important things you have going on.

If you still have too much on your plate and can't make time three days a week, then make a list of everything on your to-do list. Look at what you can automate, delegate, or eliminate. Look at what should go on your not-to-do list. Read *The 4-Hour Workweek* by Timothy Ferriss.

Ready to learn the simple version of how to get extreme results?

Maximum results in minimal time comes with eating a tighter diet, lifting weights, increasing your cardio without taking attention away from training, and enhancing what you are already doing with nutrition supplements. (We'll focus on nutrition and diet in this and the next two chapters, and then we'll discuss weight training and cardio in Part III.)

That's it in a nutshell.

It's not salads and mad runs on the treadmill, although those don't always hurt. You are not a chubby little hamster running for its life because it doesn't know what else to do.

You can't out-train a bad diet. You can be in the gym killing yourself every single day and twice a day, so proud of how much you sweat and how many calories you've burned, but if you aren't dialing in your nutrition, you are spending so much more time in the gym than you need to and not getting the results you are capable of.

Nutrition is about more than just eating a salad for lunch every day, although that may help you move forward if you are used to eating fast food every day or if your dial has been turned down pretty low. But we are talking about turning that dial to a ten. This chapter is about getting the most extreme results, not just getting healthier.

If you want to shed body fat, it's important to simply consume fewer calories than you need in a day. If you eat the same amount of calories, then you are just maintaining. If you eat a little more, that's when you can put on more muscle.

Pretty simple.

- To lose body fat means eating less calories than you burn.
- To maintain means to eat the same calories that you burn.
- To build means to eat a little more calorie than you burn.

Combining strategic weight training with strategic meal plans is how people get those drastic before-and-after pictures that most people look at and dream they could do. If you don't want to tighten up your nutrition better than what it already is, then only three hours a week in the gym won't be enough, and you'll have to work even more.

Save yourself time and math by creating an account on myfitness-pal.com and determine your calorie intake for your goal. From there, choose one of the methods below to calculate and create your own meal plan.

MACROS AND CHOOSING WHAT YOU PREFER

To get extreme results, you won't be eating salad, celery sticks, and sweating your butt off on a treadmill. You've got to think at the next level to get to the next level.

Getting extreme results is more than just eating diet food or what one would think of as health food.

One myth is that people think that just eating healthy will help them get the body of their dreams and lose a lot of weight. Sure, eating a salad instead of a burger and fries every day may help the average couch potato, but it's not gearing you toward living the high-performance life and getting the extreme results.

So if you want extreme results in minimal time, it's not eating diet food at all. It's feeding your mind, muscle, and gut what it needs to perform its best, to optimize its best, to recover its best, and to burn fat its best. Diet food does not help that.

Athletes and people with killer physiques don't eat diet food. They eat whole foods.

The truth is, there is more than just one way to approach nutrition, and I'll list a few options below to help you get your extreme results in minimal time. There isn't one way for everyone. Part of this is an adventure to discover how your body responds the best with your lifestyle while making strides toward the overall high-performance life.

If you want extreme results, you will likely have to count macro-nutrients and calories. I like the method professional bodybuilder coach John Meadows shared on his YouTube channel.

FOR MEN

Your body weight x 15 = _____ calories per day

BW x 1.25 = _____ grams of protein per day

_____ grams of protein x 4 = _____ (calories to be eaten just in protein)

BW x .4 = _____ (fat grams per day)

_____ (fat grams per day from above) x 9 = _____ (calories just from fat in a day)

(Calories from protein) _____ + (calories from fat) _____ = _____

Subtract the sum of protein and fat calories _____ from _____ (total calories from day) = _____ (calories left for carbs)

(Calories left for carbs) _____ / 4 = _____ grams of carbs for each day

Protein calories/total calories = protein macro percentage

Fat Calories/total calories = fat macro percentage

Carb calories/total calories = carb macro percentage

Note: Eating 1.25 grams of protein per pound of body weight is probably more protein in one day than you are used to. You can try calculating 0.8 grams of protein per pound of body weight to get started and work your way up to 1.25, especially if you consider yourself to be an athlete. The daily minimum recommended by the National Institute of Health is 0.36 grams per pound for a sedentary person, and athletes are usually 1 gram per pound. So the amount of protein depends on your weight, goals, and lifestyle. Professionals go up to 1.25 and even more.

After you have your protein, carbs, and fat totals for each day, you can then plug in precise measurements of food within an app like myfitnesspal.com to calculate and track. However, this particular calculation is only one way of many.

A simpler way of measuring that I personally like to use is looking at the percentages of macros and not just the grams, which is easily accessed within myfitnesspal.com as well.

If I'm not competing and still want to be lean and shredded, I keep my protein percentage to around 40 percent of total calories for the day and then choose if I'd rather have more carbs or more fat. Since I enjoy having cream in my coffee and love avocados and the healing properties of healthy fats, I prefer to have more fat than I do carbs. It's my personal preference. If there are days where I am craving rench fries, I'll calculate to make sure my fat is much lower so I can allow more carbs for that day.

More than likely, you aren't eating the numbers you thought you were. It's great to calculate every once in a while to reevaluate where you are and make adjustments but not to do on a regular basis and take attention away from the high-performance life.

Now, this is not the only way to do things. There are many ways. Part of this is that you can explore and be adventurous with your choice of macros to help you become more mindful of what you are eating so you can watch your transformation. You can even try lowering the protein a little toward 30 percent, but I personally like to keep mine higher in order to have a leaner, stronger, and sculpted physique.

I also love IFBB pro John Meadows's less-complicated way. (Sure, he's huge, but you don't have to be as big as a barn if you don't want to be!)

As a professional bodybuilder, business owner, husband, father, and man of faith, obsessing about his nutrition is that last thing he wants to do. "I have a good amount of protein, healthy carbs, just a little bit of fat, and vegetables for breakfast before going into the office. For a mid-morning snack, I have a shake with a small handful of nuts, then eat a good lunch, and then another shake and nuts for an afternoon snack. By that time, I go home for a pre-workout meal, train, and eat again right after."

If he is training to be on stage and compete with the best physiques around the world, there is much more science and counting going on, but this book isn't to help you get on stage. You can still get in phenomenal shape in minimal time.

Maybe you don't have the aspirations to physically grow to his size that wins bodybuilding championships, but you can still aspire to trim fat and sculpt your physique as you prefer for yourself.

Following these nutritional guidelines will not make you a large bodybuilder, so fear not. It takes a great deal of intentional work to get that huge anyway, my friend.

HIGH-PROTEIN MEAL PLANNING

I have found that regardless if I want more carbs or more fat, the foundation is having adequate protein.

STEP 1: CALCULATE HOW MUCH PROTEIN YOU NEED

The National Institute of Health recommends 0.36 grams of protein per pound of body weight for a sedentary person, and for an athlete, it's as high as 1 or even 1.1 grams of protein per pound of body weight. Some professionals go up to 1.25, some even more.

For fastest results, aim more for that 1 or 1.1 grams of protein per pound of body weight. Yes, that is a lot of food. If it's too much, maybe start with 0.6 and gradually increase to 0.7, then 0.8, and work your way up.

Oftentimes people see how much food they need to eat to lose fat and their response is, "Oh my gosh, I can't eat that much food!" Most people think they need to starve and eat salads every day, but that's not you. If it was, well, not anymore.

You've got to fuel your muscles, not starve them. In fact, I increase my body fat when I eat less or eat diet food. Most people do.

Your metabolism kicks in within a few weeks and you'll find yourself going from having a hard time eating that much food to actually wanting to eat more. Therefore, it's just a new habit to train yourself in to jump-start that metabolism of yours into hyperdrive. It's throwing some logs on the fire. You are training your mind and body by feeding it well, not by starving it.

If you want shape, muscle, or to be sculpted in any way, you need to feed the muscle, not starve it with salads and celery sticks.

Repeat after me: I am not a hamster.

Your muscles give you strength, burn fat, and shape your physique. So fuel them.

High-Protein Macro Breakdown Options to Choose From

- My Simple Breakdown: First, choose if you want to lose fat; then you need to be in a caloric deficit (or if you want to stay the same, or consume more to build muscle). Percentage of total calories per day: 40 percent protein, 38 percent fat, and 22 percent carbs. If you prefer carbs, then 40 percent protein, 38 percent carbs, and 22 percent fat.
- John Meadows Simple Breakdown: "I would eat breakfast, then at work at 9:30 a.m.-ish have a shake. I always kept protein powder with me that I could put in a shaker and just shake and drink. If I wanted extra calories, I would eat a handful of nuts. I would then eat lunch there or bring my own lunch. At 3:00 p.m., I would do the shake thing again! Finally, I would get home and eat a small meal, then go train, and eat a good meal after, before bed! That's the crux of it."
- John Meadows calculated formula seen below.

STEP 2: CHOOSE FAT OR CARBS

If you chose the first option above, then although the protein is the foundation, you then choose if you'd rather have fat or rather have carbs.

I already told you I prefer healthy fats. If you prefer carbs, then choose carbs as your second highest number and keep your fat low. You can introduce carb cycling to alternate and have higher carb days to look forward to, which I'll explain more later because it's more advanced.

To get a visual on how much you need to eat in a day, calculate it all in MyFitnessPal app. You can calculate it all from scratch, but again, we are looking to simplify things to save time to put toward an overall high-performing life. Getting lost in details can distract you from being more powerful in all the other important areas of life. So make it simple on yourself by just using the app, plugging in the numbers, and creating a meal plan to get your maximum results in minimal time.

If you want a formula to try, here's how John Meadows starts with his clients who are training hard. Not all formulas work for every-body, but they're great starting points to get you on track to gaining extreme results in minimal time.

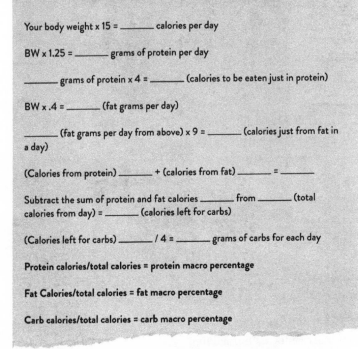

FOR MEN

Your body weight x 15 = _____ calories per day

BW x 1.25 = _____ grams of protein per day

_____ grams of protein x 4 = _____ (calories to be eaten just in protein)

BW x .4 = _____ (fat grams per day)

_____ (fat grams per day from above) x 9 = _____ (calories just from fat in a day)

(Calories from protein) _____ + (calories from fat) _____ = _____

Subtract the sum of protein and fat calories _____ from _____ (total calories from day) = _____ (calories left for carbs)

(Calories left for carbs) _____ / 4 = _____ grams of carbs for each day

Protein calories/total calories = protein macro percentage

Fat Calories/total calories = fat macro percentage

Carb calories/total calories = carb macro percentage

Take your body weight and multiply it times 15 for how many calories to eat in a day. A 220-pound man times 15 equals 3,300 calories. Protein is 1.25 grams per pound of body weight, so a 220-pound man would eat 275 grams of protein per day. With four calories in every gram of protein, that equals 1,100 calories per day just in protein. You then multiply 220 times 0.4 to get fat per day, which is 88. Multiply 88 times 9 calories per gram of fat which is 792. Adding your protein and fat calories together is 1,892 calories. Subtract 1,892 from 3,300 from the total day and you are left with 1,408 calories just for carbs. Since each carb has 4 calories per gram, dividing 1,408 by 4 equals 352 grams of carbs for each day. The macro percentages would be 1,100 divided by 3,300 equals 33 percent protein; 792 divided by 3,330 equals 24 percent fat; and 1,408 divided by 3,300 equals 43 percent carbs.

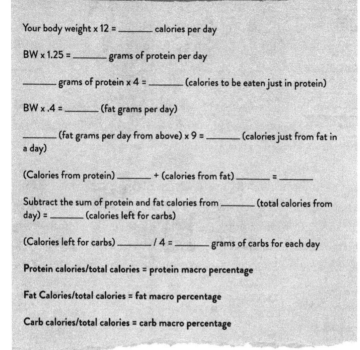

FOR WOMEN

Your body weight x 12 = _____ calories per day

BW x 1.25 = _____ grams of protein per day

_____ grams of protein x 4 = _____ (calories to be eaten just in protein)

BW x .4 = _____ (fat grams per day)

_____ (fat grams per day from above) x 9 = _____ (calories just from fat in a day)

(Calories from protein) _____ + (calories from fat) _____ = _____

Subtract the sum of protein and fat calories from _____ (total calories from day) = _____ (calories left for carbs)

(Calories left for carbs) _____ / 4 = _____ grams of carbs for each day

Protein calories/total calories = protein macro percentage

Fat Calories/total calories = fat macro percentage

Carb calories/total calories = carb macro percentage

Take your body weight and multiply it times 12 for total calories for the day. So a 155-pound female times 12 would need 1,860 calories per day. She would have 1 gram of protein per pound of body weight which would be 155 grams of protein. 155 times 4 calories per gram is 620 calories just in protein. 155 times 0.4 equals 62 grams of fat, times 9 calories per gram is 558 calories. Add protein and fat calories together and get 1,178 calories, subtract that from total calories and get 682 calories left for carbs. Divide by 4 is 171 grams of carbs. So protein breakdown would be 155 grams of protein which is 33 percent of total calories, 62 grams of fat which is 30 percent of total calories, and 170 grams of carbs which is 37 percent of total calories.

STEP 3: CREATE A MEAL PLAN BASED OFF THE MACROS YOU PREFER

I like to create my own meal plan. I find this to be simple so I can continue focusing on the high-performance life, and not just a contest-ready body.

The simplicity here is that you calculate in myfitnesspal.com, and that is your general meal plan every day, but you still switch and swap food around so you aren't bored or restricted.

For example, when it's time to eat a protein, you can switch and swap any protein you want. If you calculate 6 ounces of lean meat for lunch or dinner, you can use multiple recipes for chicken, turkey, tuna, lean steak, fish, shrimp, fat-free Greek yogurt, or a protein shake. Swap protein for protein, carb for carb, and fats for fats.

Keep it simple.

Tips to Make Meal Planning Easy

- Choose your protein, whether you are vegan, paleo, whole30, carnivore, vegetarian, and so on.
- Make it in bulk and have a few different options to choose from.
- Always keep at least two protein options in the fridge so it is easy to grab and go and is less stressful.
- Freeze some for later. Comes in handy for those extra-lazy days.
- Always have easy vegetable sides whether it's roasted vegetables, frozen, raw, steamed, or salads.
- Have containers ready to take meals with you.
- Or make it easier by hiring a meal prep service or personal chef.

Create a meal plan in advance and just eat that, swapping out foods for variety. Don't worry, it's not boring.

I like this option because I calculate 4–6 ounces of lean meat for one meal, and I'll switch out whatever lean proteins that fit that exact amount. You aren't eating the same thing every day but still have flexibility, variety, and can have more bandwidth and head-space for more important matters. And where I have a fat figured in, I'll switch fats from almond butter to creamer for my coffee, salad dressing, and so on.

Lean proteins are typically protein powders, chicken, turkey, sir-loin, salmon, tuna, fat-free plain Greek yogurt, and vegan options. If I'm having something more fatty like a roast and chicken drum-sticks, that counts as a fat, versus a chicken breast is so lean you can afford to have a fat paired with it. So often I'll eat the fattier meats because I enjoy them, but if I want to lean down more, then I'll swap for the leaner meats versus the fattier meats.

It really isn't that complicated at all.

I can blindly bring these foods with me to the studio, and if I'm traveling, it's not too hard to order a steak and a salad for a meal. If all else fails, I focus on protein and vegetables. I personally ask the server not to bring me the complimentary breadsticks because I know my weakness and would rather set myself up for success. If you put a bowl of breadsticks in front of me, I will devour them, so it's best if they just aren't there.

This enables you to be more present to succeed in all areas, not just counting macros. Do what works best for you and set yourself up for success and living a high-performance life all while becoming more and more fit.

Here is the example John did for me when we first started working together.

	FOOD	PROTEIN	CARBS	FAT	CALORIES
MEAL 1	3 organic free-range eggs (eat hard-boiled, scrambled, etc. however you want)	18	0	13.5	233
	1/2 Tbsp virgin coconut oil	0	0	7	63
	1 cup of spinach	0	0	0	0
		0	0	0	0
		0	0	0	0
		0	0	0	0
		18	0	20.5	296
MEAL 2	20 grams of whey isolate (CFM)	20	0	0	80
	1/2 cup strawberries, blueberries, or raspberries	1	10	0	44
		0	0	0	0
		21	10	0	124

	FOOD	PROTEIN	CARBS	FAT	CALORIES
MEAL 3	3 oz cooked any lean meat (turkey, chicken, or white fish)	21	0	1	93
LUNCH	1 cup of any green veggie you like	0	0	0	0
	4 oz of sweet potatoes	1	28	0	116
		0	0	0	0
		0	0	0	0
		22	28	1	209
MEAL 4	20 grams of whey isolate (CFM)	20	0	0	80
	1 Tbsp of almond butter	2	3	9	101
		0	0	0	0
		22	3	9	181
MEAL 5	3 oz cooked any lean meat (turkey, chicken, or white fish)	21	0	1	93
PRE-WORKOUT	1/2 cup (dry measure) oats	5	27	3	155
	1 Tbsp of almond butter	2	3	9	101
		0	0	0	0
		28	30	13	349

	FOOD	PROTEIN	CARBS	FAT	CALORIES
MEAL 6	3 oz cooked any lean meat (turkey, chicken, or white fish)	21	0	1	93
POST-WORKOUT	1 cup cooked white rice	4	37	0	169
		0	0	0	0
LATE SNACK	3 cups cooked air-popped popcorn	3	19	1	93
		28	56	2	355
		0	0	0	0
INTRA-WORKOUT	Mag 10: 2 scoops	20	11	0	127
		0	0	0	0
		20	11	0	127
		0	0	0	0
TOTALS					
		159	138	45.5	
CALORIES		x4	x4	x9	
PERCENT OF TOTAL CALORIES		636	552	410	1,598
		40%	35%	26%	

Pre-workout meal (one to three hours prior to training): any lean meat or protein at least the size of your palm, cupped palm size of a carb, and a thumb size of fat.

Intra-workout drink with essential aminos.

Post-workout meal (forty-five to sixty minutes after training):

any lean meat or protein, fast-absorbing carb like white rice, and a thumb size of fat. Don't forget vegetables.

Lean protein examples: turkey, fish, flank steak, shrimp, fat-free plain Greek yogurt.

Carb examples: white potato, sweet potato, Japanese purple potato, brown rice, brown rice pasta, old-fashioned or rolled oats, white rice or cream of rice (better as post-workout), natural jelly without added sugar to add to Greek yogurt, fruit, quinoa.

Fat examples: extra virgin olive oil, high-grade fish oil in capsules, nut butters, MCT oil (stimulates more fat loss), grass-fed butter, full-fat cream. Omit any seed oils, which are in most salad dressings.

WHY IT WORKS

With this method, you aren't being obsessed, but you are being mindful. Obsession is when you have to calculate all day when you eat or drink something, distracting from the more important things in life. Your mind, health, marriage, or kids doesn't need that obsession. If you want to kill your passion, then feed your obsession.

We want to make this as simple as possible to get the results that you want, which means the health and body you want as well as the lifestyle. I find it pointless to waste time overcalculating when I would rather increase quality in every area of life, not just my diet.

Calculate once or twice to get a good idea of what you should be eating, swap out foods that are similar, and reevaluate to make sure you are keeping yourself up to those standards. After a while of not calculating, you may find that your protein has slipped far below your needs to have lower body fat, that you have been eating too much, or not eating enough. It's a great way to keep yourself in check but not daily unless you really are training to be on a stage or in a muscle magazine.

TIMING YOUR MEALS FOR POWERED PERFORMANCE, RECOVERY, AND TRANSFORMATION

The most important meals take place before, during, and after your training session. You need to be powered well and to refuel well. Your muscles need to be fed and refueled. If you aren't eating enough, for example, you may struggle to get in the ideal workout you have the potential to do, therefore cutting yourself short to what you are truly capable of.

Center meals around your protein, and then center those around your workouts.

PRE-WORKOUT MEAL

Try to eat one to three hours prior to training so your energy is going into training and not into digestion. Have your protein, carb, and a tiny bit of fat. If you have a fattier meat, then omit the fat.

If eating three hours before training feels like too long of a time without food and you find yourself lacking energy for your workout, then try two hours.

I love eating and want to eat often, so I prefer eating about one hour before. I don't care to wait any longer! While for others, they may think it's too close to their workout. Find what's best for you and don't overcomplicate it; stick within the one to three hours prior to training.

INTRA-WORKOUT MEAL

This is the supplements you start sipping on a few minutes before training to get into your bloodstream. Drink during the workout. This is where I love drinking essential aminos.

POST-WORKOUT MEAL

John Meadows loves to eat forty-five to sixty minutes after training and the best time to have your fast-absorbing carbs like white rice, paired with protein, and a little bit of fat to help digestion.

HOW TO DO CARB CYCLING TO GET EXTREME RESULTS

Carb cycling can be a great way of shedding some body fat and tightening up your physique, whether it's for a challenge, a body-building competition, vacation, or an event. A few weeks to a month before an event, carb cycling can be a magical tool to get the results you want, even if not counting calories or macros.

Now, to be honest, I personally didn't use carb cycling for figure competitions because I've always gotten myself lean enough that I didn't need to. Many competitors do it a few weeks prior to a show to get leaner and add fullness to their muscles and shape. You can use this for an extra edge for your own results, too.

For carb cycling to work, you'll need to be in a calorie deficit already and then on certain days reintroduce carbs.

Carb cycling is fun to experiment with, from higher carb days that's best for training days, medium-carb days (which would be your normal amount of carbs), and then low-carb days where your carbs are lower than your normal amount. You can experiment how many days for each, like maybe starting with two days low carb, then three days normal carb, and two days high carb.

Or maybe try three low-carb days, then three normal-carb days, and one high-carb day. Experiment and see how you feel and how your body responds.

It's a tool to help you transform and the transformation doesn't ever end. You can keep building, experimenting, transforming and having fun with it.

Something to love about this method is that obviously being in a calorie deficit makes you hungry, but the light at the end of the tunnel is that you have more carbs to reload and feel amazing. You have those carbs to look forward to and you don't feel deprived.

The plus side is that you'll have low days, but then you will have medium and high days to be looking forward to and excited about. So for some people, they feel like they are "dieting" only one or two days a week, when they are on low-carb days.

Another benefit is that when you are on the hunt for fat loss and need to be in a calorie deficit to get there, carb cycling can help you from yo-yo dieting.

Save those reload or high-carb days specifically for your training days for energy and to refuel after your workouts. For example, I try to group all my heavy training days in the beginning of the week, so therefore those are the same days I'll have high carbs. And then at the end of the week, I'll go low or medium carbs when it's either an off day or an active rest day. By the time Monday comes around for training legs, my body is soooooo ready for those carbs again!

This really revs up the metabolism, energy, and filling out muscles for more shape rather than the days you are on low-carb days.

HIGH-CARB DAYS OR CARB-RELOAD DAY

I used my training days, which were usually Monday, Tuesday, and Wednesday, for my high-carb days, which meant I literally doubled the amount of carbs I typically ate. Very specifically one to three hours prior to training and forty-five to sixty minutes after training, then another meal with double carbs.

Choose the training days you want the most energy, and use those two or three days for high-carb days. This means you double the amount of carbs you normally eat specifically for your pre-workout and post-workout meal so your body utilizes that fuel most efficiently.

Remember, as a high performer, everything needs to be strategically efficient to perform higher in every area.

MEDIUM-CARB DAYS (NORMAL CARBS)

Thursday and Friday were medium-carb days, which was my basic day, just normal carbs. I even played around with taking out the medium-carb days and only doing high-carb and low-carb days just to experiment.

After your two or three days of high-carb days, then lower your carbs back down to your normal amount for two to three days.

LOW-CARB DAYS

After your medium-carb days or also known as your normal-carb days, then lower carbs more for another two or three days. You will be hungry, like you are dieting, but no worries because you have a high-carb day to look forward to, so hang in there! Your body will then eat up those high carbs and that's the moment you'll look and feel your best.

For me, Saturday and Sunday were low-carb days, where I didn't have anything starchy but just vegetables and maybe one small serving of fruit. Even then, I usually kept the fruit out just for those two days. By the time Monday rolled around to train legs, my body was READY to eat up those carbs and not store it as fat.

To give you an extreme example of this, I can show you how I made a huge mistake. I was experimenting with my carbs for NPC Figure Nationals in Fort Lauderdale. I kept my carbs really low and was new at all of this. My physique was not at its best while I was on stage against the best physiques around the nation.

After stepping off stage, I had more carbs and wine to celebrate that I was done, even if it was not my best. Later that night, I took off my dress and my muscles ate those carbs and had the physique I needed on stage. My muscles were round, shapely, full, and even appeared more lean and sculpted. Before the carbs, I was really lean but looked deflated. After the carbs, muscles were more full and defined.

That's an extreme example of what carb cycling can do. When you have days of lower carbs and then introduce the carb cycling and higher carbs, you transform from deflated shape to a full and sculpted shape.

Try it sometime, and see how your body responds, especially after doing this for a while. The leaner you get, the more noticeable the changes are.

ENHANCING RECOVERY, RESULTS, AND PERFORMANCE WITH NUTRITION SUPPLEMENTS

An overweight and sedentary customer named Jerome came to me and said he bought some natural fat burners off my website. He said, "If someone like Bailey would recommend them, then they must work!"

Yes, they work, but only if you are working also. They enhance what you are already doing; they can't enhance nothing.

Jerome didn't do any work or make lifestyle changes for the fat burners to do any good.

For those fat burners to really help, he needed to be doing some sort of exercise, like swimming, yoga, or Pilates, while also improving his nutrition. (I am convinced weight training will give you the ultimate transformation, but if you don't like it or don't want to, it's better to find something to move versus doing nothing at all!)

Supplements are extremely helpful to enhance what you are

already doing with your training and nutrition, but don't count on them doing all the work. (And always check with your doctor.)

Get moving and eat better. Your health depends on it.

Once you get into a healthier rhythm, then it makes some sense to enhance your training and nutrition. I personally focus on recovery and essential aminos while I am training to refuel my muscles, hinder muscle breakdown, and repair my muscles.

I'm less sore; it makes me more mindful that I am fueling my body; and I can see the changes. Whereas if I just took supplements without behavior change, there would be hardly any change at all.

So for extreme results in minimal time, choose a diet style that works best for you without taking away from your high-performance life and enhance it with nutrition supplements.

EXTREME RESULTS CALL FOR EXTREME CARE

Be smart. If you haven't been working out at all and want to turn this dial from a zero to a ten, you can do it, but you have to be smart and listen to your body (and your doctor, of course).

You don't want to fall in the pattern of turning that dial up to a hard ten instead of easing into it and causing yourself so much injury and harm that you can't move, get burned out, or defeated and end up turning that dial back to zero again.

You can still get that dial to a ten, but be cautious. Don't lift more weight than what is safe. You can be a ten without harming yourself. Be impeccable about form, breathing techniques, stretching, physical therapy for prevention, heat and ice as needed, massages, chiropractic, acupuncture, or whatever you need to keep your body recovering and performing well.

Drink lots of water, take really great care of your gut health to optimize absorption and brain health as well.

You can even use supplements to help restore your muscles and supplements to help fight inflammation and joint health.

If you want your body and life to perform like a race car, you've gotta pit it and restore it often so it can continue doing so.

You have to remember that professional athletes can perform at that level for such extended periods of time not only because of the training but because of the self-care and treatment as well. So can you. And you should.

Start asking yourself things you could do to help your own mind and body recover and perform better, to train better the next day. For some, they love cryotherapy; others love massage. Think of one thing you can do that keeps your car on the track to the high-performance life.

KEY TAKEAWAY

By following this chapter, you are capable of getting in the best shape of your life in only three days a week. Four days if you really want to get wild and it doesn't take away from the other areas of your life.

You need to be emotionally healthy, spiritually healthy, relationally healthy with spouse, family, friends, and community. You still need to have dreams, goals, adventures, and hobbies. If you pour your entire life into fitness and counting macros, the other areas might suffer, taking you further away from the high-performance life.

Don't make it complicated.

As a high performer, you have many areas you want to excel in—areas that take time, focus, and clarity. Instead of spending excessive hours in the gym, bring your attention to what other areas in your life that could use awareness or joy to help your overall performance.

HIGH-PERFORMANCE EXERCISE

1. Choose your macros or method from above and write out your own meal plan. Interchange proteins for proteins, carbs for carbs, and fats for fats so you aren't bored, yet not obsessing about tracking every morsel each day.

2. We will talk about weightlifting more in Part III, but to give you an overview, you should lift three days a week targeting the largest muscle groups for faster fat burn and transformation. Add a fourth training day if you really want to for a lagging body part and if your life allows for a fourth training day.

3. After a week or two of getting used to training three days a week as a priority, then introduce one day of HIIT. Slowly increase HIIT to two to three days. Do either after training back or chest day, or on off days. Add abs and calves just once a week. (Again, this will be discussed more in upcoming chapters.)

4. Keep nutrition before, during, and after training your most important meals, and let the other meals and protein shakes fall in place around it.

5. Use supplements to fuel, recover, and help burn fat.

6. Carb cycle the last two to three weeks or so of your training program or leading up to an event to scorch even more body fat and more extreme results!

7. Basic rule for your nutrition goals is that if you want to lose fat, then eat less calories than you burn. If you want to stay the same, then eat the same. If you want more muscle or to put on more weight, then eat more. Get extreme results without making any of this more complicated.

8. Set yourself up for success. Rest, self-care, set up your renewal rhythms we discussed in earlier chapters and surround yourself with like-minded people. Don't neglect the other areas of your life. Either cook in bulk or hire meal prep service so it is accessible to you. Drink plenty of water throughout the day too, and be sure to get in all your meals even if you are too busy. Feed the muscles; don't starve them.

9. Be your own best cheerleader and coach in your own mind. Build yourself up; don't rely on others for that. When training, make every repetition better than the last, especially when you get tired. Dig deep and keep yourself challenged without hurting or injuring yourself.

10. Use this method to get extreme results in minimal time. In the next chapter, we can learn how to maintain it for longevity, sustainability, and lifestyle for the high-performance life. You can then learn how to adjust and be a little less extreme while still accomplishing your goals.

11. If you had nine extra hours per week, where and what could you do with them? Refer to your ten areas and your goals for each area.

CHAPTER 6

HOW TO GET LEAN WITHOUT BEING EXTREME

I was at the doctor's office after one of my competitions. I'd mentioned on my last visit that I'd be competing, so the doctor asked how I did and to see my contest pictures.

I brought out my phone to show him a stage photo and his eyes widened. He looked up at me, then back at my phone in a bit of shock, and said, "Do you realize you accomplished in six months what people train for ten years to do?"

This happened less than two years after I crushed both of my ankles and had to learn to walk all over again. Healing was absolutely crucial before tackling this big goal of competing, but the awesome part that I later realized is that it doesn't need to be as complicated as people make it.

I've already gotten extremely lean. I've been there and done that; won some trophies with it. None of it was easy, especially with my weight-gaining hypothyroid disease and doing it without drugs or fat burners, but it wasn't complicated.

I was that lean because I treated it as a sport, and I lived that sport. Maybe someday, I'll get extreme again.

"Why would you ever compete again?" my functional medicine doctor asked as we were correcting the thyroid imbalances in my body.

I looked down, searching for my answer.

"Well, maybe I'll get back into it just so I can keep my credibility and authority in the health and fitness industry. I want to be able to truly help people, and having people's trust helps me to better help them."

He shot back, "You already have that credibility and authority, and you never need to step on stage again. Believe me, even if you never step on stage again, you have all the credibility in the world."

The comment meant a lot, coming from this deeply respected physician who worked with professional athletes internationally.

I was deeply humbled to have his respect and blessings to teach you exactly how I do it and how to adjust your own dial to be as extreme as you want but while keeping the most important things in life where they need to be: a priority.

NO NEED TO BE EXTREME

So you are looking for more balanced nutrition, perhaps needing to lower the dial on intensity a little bit, and you still want to make progress? The good news is that you can.

Let's first get through any kind of sugarcoating here, though: with the combination of better nutrition and workouts, you will be able to get the results you are looking for. The tighter the nutrition and workouts, the tighter the results you'll get. It's that simple.

It's not easy, but it's simple.

Don't make nutrition harder than what it needs to be to get the results that you want. With a little less intense approach and not as extreme transformation, you can still make progress toward your goal in a much more sustainable way through these nutrition tips.

What a relief to know you don't need to do extreme dieting or waste crazy time in the gym to get the lean and strong physique you want.

As a high performer, you constantly seek to improve and perform higher in every area of life, and to do that requires an effective strategy. It means being on your A game with the important things, but you can't move forward if you try to be on your A game with absolutely everything or you'll fall apart. You've got to remember the things on your not-to-do list.

You'll burn the candle from both ends and from the middle while you are at it. I'm sure you have felt it and seen it in others.

You'll crash and burn, be exhausted, and turn to survival mode where that candle burning turns into destroying everything you have worked for. Your marriage is falling apart, you keep putting off your health, you keep putting off the gym, and positive relationships that you really need in your life are dissolving.

This book isn't about survival mode and low performance; this is about being a high performer so you can live your best life with the best health. It's okay to look back at your dial and adjust it. You don't have to live at a ten all the time, like the advice from the last chapter was geared toward. Reevaluate to see if this is a time to dial back to a nine or an eight. A little lower if you need to. I know there have been times in my life when I have.

It's better to adjust that dial lower, rather than turning it down to a zero and jumping off the ship completely.

The key is an effective strategy. With your own dial, you can adjust your strategy so you improve as a high performer in all areas.

Some seasons you may be at a ten (like getting ready for a special event, beach vacation, wedding, cruise, or even a competition), but when you prefer to dial it back and be less extreme with your nutrition, you can still make progress all around or maintain your hard work.

This is the chapter on how to maintain all of your hard work. You can also use this if starting off extreme and pedal to the metal like in the last chapter. You can most certainly ease into it gradually making improvements each day.

SITTING DOWN WITH THE LEGEND HIMSELF

I was at a point that I was doing well in figure competitions, including finishing in the top five against some of the best physiques around the world at the Arnold Amateur in Columbus. I was already strong and lean, but I wanted to better understand nutrition.

I wanted to know why my trainer would allow me to eat only half an apple with twelve raw almonds. I wanted to know why I ate certain things at certain times. I craved to learn and understand.

The more I talked with professionals in the industry, the more they referred me to John Meadows.

I know I've already told you about him, but at the time, all I knew was that he was the guy that muscle magazines interviewed; professional athletes and celebrities hired him; he formulated his own supplements; owned his own company; people called him a genius; and here, we worked out at the same gym and I didn't even know him.

Someone pointed him out in the café of the gym one day and I gathered my courage and curiosity to ask him, "What do I need to do to know what you know and do what you do?"

There's no way to answer that quickly after decades of his experience, but I offered to organize seminars for him to make it worth his time. I eagerly wanted to know what he knew. I was tired of training six days a week and sometimes twice a day and eating so few calories.

He took me under his wing.

The moment I sat down with John Meadows, it seemed like the heavens of training, nutrition, and longevity had fallen upon me.

I realized that it does not need to be complicated at all, but most of us make it that way—including most personal trainers whom we have all hired.

Most of us make things so complicated that we don't follow through. We overthink it and over-research it, which paralyzes us even more.

IMAGINE WHAT YOU ARE CAPABLE OF WITHOUT MAKING EVERYTHING SO COMPLICATED AND PARALYZING.

I know almost everything I've done in the past was complicated with not many results. I did the fad diets, fat burners, and worked out five to six days a week and seemed to only get skinny fat, frustrated, and hungry.

There was of course more that I needed to understand and to make changes.

We sat down and John drew pictures on scrap pieces of paper in the gym's café, explaining the importance of nutrition timing and the glycogen transporters that feed the carbs from the bloodstream into the muscle, and the small window of time that it's best to have carbs for better results. Of course, there is contrary research just like anything else, but by decades of his own success and his clients' success, as they say, the proof is in the pudding.

He took my physique to more transformation without drugs, extreme work, or extreme diets. It all came down to simplifying training and nutrition. I actually discovered how to train less, do less cardio, and eat more food.

Work smarter, not just harder.

THE SIMPLE WAY TO PORTION CONTROL WITHOUT COUNTING CALORIES

Food and nutrition go much further than just losing body fat and going on a diet. It is what fuels your body and your mind and can empower you to take steps that are much simpler than you think.

The simplest way to get extreme results guides you to calculate macros only once and create a meal plan for yourself to hit your goals, as I shared in the last chapter. You calculate it once, and simply swap out the proteins for proteins, carbs for carbs, and fats for fats. It's a great way to get fast results while eating wholesome food.

But if you don't want to calculate at all, the much simpler way is to use your hand to determine your portions.

Dr. John Berardi of Precision Nutrition established the gold standard of being able to do so, where instead of calculating with a scale and your face isn't lost in your phone tracking every morsel while life goes on by, you can eyeball your meals.

Yes, you still need to be mindful of what you eat. You can't just eat what you want mindlessly and expect a positive change.

I got started into bodybuilding competitions and had very strict diets following very strict meal plans. Although meal plans and strict diets are great for competitors and professional athletes, it's not something realistic or sustainable for the rest of the world.

I eventually tried flexible dieting where you can eat anything you want as long as it fits into your macros for the day. I hated that more than anything else. Some absolutely love it and swear by it, but I just hated it. It was time consuming and annoying to sit there and calculate every gram to eat that day.

What I found that worked better than anything else when it came to balancing nutrition while not obsessing about it was following the golden standards of Precision Nutrition's portion guide by simply using your hand to measure portions.

Your hand is always with you, which makes for a perfect tool to measure your meals. I've used this same approach to dial in my body fat even lower by carb cycling. We'll talk more about that a little later in this section, but the point is, unless you are about to step on a stage, mastering this will help you with all the muscle gains or fat loss you want to make!

This method has been the easiest for me when maintaining in the off season without counting calories.

Cover model Jamie Eason uses the same Precision Nutrition approach from *Oxygen* magazine challenges. Here's how to do it:

- **Portion Control for Men:** Choose a leaner protein the size of your palm, and double it. Have two fist-sized portions of vegetables, two small cupped hands of a carb, and two thumb sizes of fats. Eating three to four meals like this is about 2,300–3,000 calories, so there is a lot of wiggle room to make adjustments to see how your body is best responding.
- **Portion Control for Women:** Use one palm size for a protein, one fist size for vegetables, one small cupped hand for carbs,

and one thumb size for fats. Eating three to four meals like this would be between 1,200 and 1,500 calories per day.

Examples of Protein: meat, fish, eggs (the yolk would count as a fat), cottage cheese, non-fat plain Greek yogurt, protein shakes (whey, casein, plant based).

Vegetables: frozen, fresh, steamed, roasted, stir fried, or raw. Broccoli, spinach, salad, asparagus, cucumber, greens, etc.

Carbs: oats, pasta, beans, and fruit.

Fats: oils (not vegetable or seed oils), extra virgin olive oil, extra virgin coconut oil in dark containers, grass-fed butter, nut butters, nuts, and seeds.

This is a great way to start, but here are some guidelines on how to make changes if you need more or less food to get to your goals.

You May Need More Food if You:

- Are larger
- Still feel really hungry
- Eat less frequently throughout the day
- Are much more active
- Want to add bulk or put on muscle

If that's the case, you can tweak it to add a little more protein or another thumb size of fat. If wanting more muscle, then add another cupped handful of carbs specifically forty-five minutes to sixty minutes after training.

You May Need Less Food if You:

- Are smaller to begin with
- Feel too full
- Eat more frequently during the day
- Are less active
- Are trying to lose weight

If that's the case for you, then you can tweak by removing some carbs or a fat from your day and continue to readjust. Just make sure carbs are before and after training; those are the most important meals of the day.

PRE-WORKOUT MEAL

This is where you have a meal anywhere between one hour and three hours prior to training. I find this one important to fuel my workouts. Without it, I can feel the difference in my energy, strength, and focus. If I'm feeling weak for a workout, it's pretty simple that my workout won't be as good as it could be, therefore having less-than-optimal results.

Fuel yourself to make the most of your nutrition and training so you can get the results you want in less time, so you can focus on the more important things in life.

If you eat too soon before training, then your energy goes to your stomach to digest it instead of the results and strength you are focusing on. You want your meal before training already digesting and in your bloodstream.

My favorite pre-workout meal is similar to the Precision Nutrition gold standard. I'll have one palm size of protein and one cupped handful of carbs, which is usually old-fashioned oatmeal or a sweet potato for me. If I have a fatty meat like roast or chicken thigh, then I won't add fat. If it's a lean protein like chicken breast or a tuna pack, then add a thumb size of fat. It's that simple. If I am carb cycling and it's a high-carb day, then I double the carbs. If it's a low-carb day, then I don't have the carbs.

INTRA-WORKOUT

I am a big believer in supplements. Our earth doesn't contain the nutrients it once did, plus supplements enhance what you are already doing. I'll use supplements for health, wellness, gut health, brain health, joint health, decreasing inflammation in the body, vitamins, as well as my performance and recovery.

Some take supplements without making changes to their diet or training, and they wonder why the supplements don't work, but the work is up to you. Supplements only enhance what you are already doing. Take Jerome, my example from Chapter 5. He didn't change a thing with his diet or exercise, yet he took fat burners expecting big change. It just doesn't work like that.

I used to do that before I knew any better. I wasn't eating a healthy diet or training very smart as a teen or even in my twenties, but I took fat burners so I wouldn't get fat. Neither smart nor healthy. Now I train smarter and eat more. What's even better is that I don't fear getting fat because I have the understanding of all that I'm sharing with you. I live, eat, and train like a high performer, not like a fearful teenager anymore.

What is in your nutrition goes into your bloodstream, and then it goes into your muscles when training. John explained it in a much more scientific way as he drew the glycogen transporters opening up from the bloodstream into the muscles on the scrap piece of paper that day, but what matters most is not only understanding what he said but doing it. Wait too long to get the nutrients into the bloodstream and those glycogen transporters close, and your muscles won't absorb it. Instead, they could store it as fat.

The more we talk and don't do, the more opportunities close, just like those glycogen transporters. They are open for a small window of time to take advantage of. You understand opportunities; this is another one but for nutrition to make your physique goals.

John has been working with supplement companies for years, and he has started his own supplement company. Being the honest and ethical man that he is, I trust his work and use his supplements where I can further enhance the nutrition and training that I am already doing, no matter if my dial is at a two or a ten.

POST-WORKOUT MEAL

After a workout, those glycogen transporters are still open, and this is the best time to consume those fast-absorbing carbohydrates like white rice, pancakes, and burgers. I try to eat mine forty-five to sixty minutes after training to make sure those muscles are getting fed well in the right amount of time for max results.

Again, I still use the Precision Nutrition way to have one palm-size protein, cupped handful of fast-absorbing carbs, and a thumb size of fat if I don't have a fatty meat. Sometimes I'll allow myself to have double the carbs as if I was carb cycling.

Picture yourself as a glycogen tank when you are working out. You want that tank full but not overflowing. Anything overflowing could turn into fat and not get absorbed into your system.

For some reason, when people want to get in great shape, they'll snack on an apple or celery before or after their workout thinking that trick will work, but there is no tricking the body. The trick is in your mind to learn how to feed the body what it needs in order to fuel what you want it to do and become. It takes more than celery sticks, sweetheart.

CHOOSE QUALITY FOOD FOR A QUALITY BODY, GUT, AND BRAIN

Our bodies are made to digest and absorb the nutrients we eat. That means you are what your body has absorbed; so quality does matter.

As John would say, "You are what you have eaten, has eaten." So eat high-quality food like cage-free eggs and grass-fed beef.

You want wholesome and micronutrient-rich foods to keep you fueled and healthy going down to the cellular level.

There is a thing called inflammatory foods, and they do exactly that: inflame you. Some foods contribute to an inflammatory response in the body, to where the body and mind cannot function its best, heal, or recover very quickly. Endless studies show how sugar contributes to such inflammation, and it feeds yeast in the body that creates this candida epidemic that has been found to be the root of many diseases and disorders.

One statistic shows that one in every three people have some sort of food intolerance. The more you put something in your body that isn't tolerable, the more it continues to build an inflamed environment within you.

Thriving health and vitality is almost impossible in inflamed environments, so being able to identify those stressors in your body to eliminate them can help create a better environment where your metabolism can work in your favor versus the opposite.

Ask your doctor for allergy tests to determine food allergens and sensitivities. Once I learned that my body cannot tolerate gluten, eggs, and dairy, I removed them and found optimal options for my absorption and increased energy and clarity.

CARB CYCLING WITHOUT COUNTING CALORIES AND MACROS AND GETTING BETTER RESULTS

There are a few different ways to carb cycle, down to counting each macronutrient, but if you have known me for a while, I'm obsessed to find measurable ways without having to track calories and macros obsessively. Let's get our faces out of our phones every once in a while and pay attention to living, all while making progress at the same time, right?

If prepping for a show or a professional athlete, you will need to track them then, but when not prepping, I've found it's crucial to give your mind and body a break and put time and focus elsewhere for that high-performance life.

Just as you have customized a great meal plan for yourself for your own goals, you can still carb cycle for even greater results without counting a single calorie.

NORMAL CALORIE DEFICIT BEFORE CARB CYCLING STARTS

I found the meal plan that worked best for me was tweaked from the Precision Nutrition guidelines to have a lean protein the size of my palm, a fat the size of my thumb, veggies to fill me, and then I would have only two or three servings of carbs each day. The carbs were the size of a cupped handful.

I ate two or three meals like that, and then two snacks were protein shakes with at least 20 grams of protein, and coupled with either a thumb size of fat, or about one-fourth cup berries.

I was very specific about my carb timing, as I've learned from coach and bodybuilding legend John Meadows IFBB Pro. The most important meals of the day are your pre-workout meal one to three hours before training, a carb while training like Intra-Carb from Granite Supplements along with essential aminos, and then the post-workout meal forty-five to sixty minutes after training.

I am religious to timing my meals around my workouts because it contributes to the best progress, energy, strength, and recovery.

WHEN READY TO START CARB CYCLING

There are many ways to play with carb cycling, and like I said, I focus on ways to make progress without having to count every macro or calorie. The method I did was pretty simple.

I'm all about making things less complicated than what they need to be so you can still make progress while enjoying what matters most in life.

Once I've established a healthy calorie deficit with my three meals and two shakes, I referred to that as my medium-carb day, all while keeping the protein the same.

HIGH-CARB DAYS OR CARB-"RELOAD" DAYS

I used my training days, which were usually Monday, Tuesday, and Wednesday, for my high-carb days, which meant I literally doubled the amount of carbs I typically ate. Very specifically one to three hours prior to training and forty-five to sixty minutes after training; then another meal with double carbs, and then my two protein shakes. So if I ate a cupped handful of cooked old-fashioned oats for my carbs prior to training, then I would double that carb and double all the other carbs in each meal for each high-carb day.

MEDIUM-CARB DAYS (NORMAL CARBS)

Thursday and Friday were medium-carb days, which was my basic day, just with normal carbs. I even played around with taking out the medium-carb days and only doing high-carb and low-carb days just to experiment.

LOW-CARB DAYS

Saturday and Sunday were low-carb days where I didn't have anything starchy, but I just ate vegetables and maybe one small serving of fruit. Even then, I usually eliminated the fruit for those two days. By the time Monday rolled around to train legs, my body was ready to eat up those carbs and not store it as fat.

CARB CYCLE WEEK EXAMPLE

Monday: High-carb day. Double the amount of carbs. Train legs.

Tuesday: High-carb day. Double the amount of carbs. Train chest, shoulders, and triceps for an hour. Do about twenty minutes of HIIT after training.

Wednesday: High-carb day. Double the amount of carbs. Train back and biceps. Do about twenty minutes of HIIT after training.

Thursday: Medium-carb day. Normal amount of carbs on my meal plan.

Friday: Medium-carb day. Normal amount of carbs on my meal plan.

Saturday: Low-carb day. Remove or lower carbs and focus on protein, fats, and vegetables. Body will eat up carbs by Monday to train again.

Sunday: Low-carb day. Remove or lower carbs and focus on protein, fats, and vegetables. Body will eat up carbs by Monday to train again.

Those are the basic rules I follow when I'm not training and dieting to a ten and not trying to be a ten.

I struggled a great deal with this after I had an emergency

C-section and was patiently waiting to heal so I could be active again. I've been winning figure competitions, and my identity was being lean, ripped, and recognized by bodybuilding.com as their top twenty physiques.

I became determined to get lean and strong again, but this time I did it without counting calories or macros every day. I made sure I kept my protein about 40 percent of my total for the day. I had an idea of what that looked like, so each day I made sure I ate that much no matter the protein sources as long as it was ethical and could interchange the proteins, carbs, and fats.

I was mindful every day but not obsessed.

Some would say it was because of genetics, but if you look at my genetics, that would actually count against me. I have more obesity and health problems in my family, including the fact I have the notorious Hashimoto's and hypothyroid disease with the slow metabolism and lethargy symptoms. I have to conquer more than what people realize. It's just as easy for me to put on fat as it is to lose it, but it requires the minimum of higher protein.

So now that you are empowered to adjust your own dial for your own intensity, you can still be mindful of your meals and make progress without being extreme about it.

It's a much more balanced approach where you can still make progress and maintain all of your hard work. But this means preparing more food than what you were probably expecting, and this can overwhelm you. Let's make that even simpler so you can have your meals done in record time while living the high-performance life. Chapter 7 shows you how.

KEY TAKEAWAY

It's okay to dial back and enjoy life a little more, laugh more, breathe more, and not freak out because you had an extra serving of mashed potatoes.

The amount of discipline and obsession it takes to be at a ten ultimately risks taking energy from other areas of your life you wish to perform better. When you are stuck in your phone calculating every single ounce, gram, and morsel you put into your body, your child has already grown, your marriage has dissolved, or life just passed you by.

There's a time and a place to be a ten, but it's at a great cost. It's when you need to reflect and ask what matters most.

Truthfully, you can have a strong, lean, and ripped body while not striving to be a ten or being extreme. You can do it without calculating your macros every day. Sure, sometimes you may need to reevaluate and tweak some things but not to the point of ruining the quality of your life, health, and relationships.

HIGH-PERFORMANCE EXERCISE

1. Continue lifting three days a week, and adjust intensity if you'd like. Adjust the dial to wherever you want it.
2. Customize your own meal plan by using your hand (if you're not using a calculated meal plan from the last chapter). Tweak as needed for your own body and goals. Action: Write down your meal plan if you haven't already.
3. (Optional) Carb cycle two to three weeks before your event to get even better results without counting.

4. Continue to time your carbs one to three hours before a workout and forty-five minutes to sixty minutes after.

5. You are what you absorb, so choose wholesome foods and supplements.

CHAPTER 7

THE SIMPLEST NUTRITION TO GET IN THE BEST SHAPE OF YOUR LIFE

In college, I was absolutely clueless about how to eat. Even though I set records, I still wonder how fast of a sprinter I could have been if I'd only understood this simple nutrition.

I was at my heaviest weight and starved myself because my immature thinking was that the bigger I was, the slower I would be. I still remember being in tears in the athletic trainers' room, when the coach coldly said, "Yeah, you are one of the bigger ones," and walked away.

So I starved myself even more. I ran extra miles, trained up and down the McKinley Monument stairs in Canton, Ohio—108 stairs to get to the top. I did it over and over again until I couldn't anymore. I was determined to just keep running to run off the fat and get faster. I didn't know any better how absurd it was to not figure in rest, recovery, and proper nutrition.

For spring break, the top performers in each event got on a bus to train with the Dallas Cowboys and Olympic Gold Medalist training partners in the Florida Gators Stadium. We usually didn't stop for meals but made the most out of snacks from gas stations. Hooray for lots of Pop-Tarts.

While our busload of track and field athletes took over the gas station to pay for our sugary snacks, one of our nationally ranked distance runners mumbled out of concern, "How are we supposed to eat healthy? You'd think a blueberry muffin would be healthy, but it has forty-nine carbs."

She had very evident six-pack abs, so she obviously knew what she was talking about. I, on the other hand, was enjoying my Pop-Tart and wondered, "What the hell is a carb?"

We eventually gas stationed and muffin-carbed our way to Florida. For our first run, the coach gathered us around the base of Gators' stadium. He looked up to the top of the stadium in the blazing sun and told us to run all the way up to the top and back down—seven times.

"I don't care if you run, walk, or crawl...seven times. Go!"

By the end, my legs were shaking so bad that they were vibrating off the stands. But just to be clear, I beat everyone, even the guys. That was a super-proud moment for me.

I then tore my Achilles' tendon while hurdling on the track and had to redshirt that year. So I started working more hours in the school's weight room as a trainer and spotter.

I remember days just hanging with some of my favorite people: the baseball and football players. And not even for sexual reasons or for any kind of attention, but because I honestly just liked being one of the guys.

Eventually, we all grew up and pursued different dreams.

More than twenty years later, one of the guys reached out to me to ask for help with his training and nutrition.

We shared our aches and pains of overcoming and recovering from 2020 as business owners and the stress it put on us all. Talking about depression, mental health, marriage, family, and trusting God.

You know, the important things.

I gave him a bullet-point version of this entire book, and he ran with it. He started with the nuts and bolts of training the larger muscle groups about three days a week. He made sure he was eating at least 1 gram of protein per pound of body weight. When I told him that, he was shocked because he wasn't even eating half of that.

I responded, "Losing weight usually means eating more of the right food (a shit ton of protein!) and not starving or restricting so much. I mean, you can't go crazy and eat what you want of course, but calculate how many grams of protein you need in a day, and divide that among three or six meals (whatever works for your lifestyle). Then eat a good fat the size of your thumb and lots of vegetables. Maybe a meal or two can have a cupped handful of carbs or more depending on how you respond to carbs."

"You just spoke my language!" said my ol' tobacco-chewing football player friend.

Only two and a half months later, he reached out again to say this lifestyle had completely changed his life. He had lost thirty-six pounds and was down three pant sizes. He almost had six-pack abs without even training abs, and he was healthier, with perfect blood pressure, perfect cholesterol, no more arthritis pain, and an overabundance of energy.

He is now in the best shape of his life besides when he was a full-time boxer training constantly. But now he's a business owner, father, husband, and man of faith. And I am really proud of him.

NUTRITION IS MORE THAN JUST EATING HEALTHY TO LOSE FAT AND GET IN SHAPE

If you are eating pizza and snacks and drinking Coke and lattes every day, then maybe it would be a benefit to just have the baby step of a goal to just be healthier. But this book is geared more toward high performers who want more than just being a little healthier.

They want to be their absolute best in every area of life, including being in the best shape.

This means following some sort of meal plan, whether it's macros, a simpler way like John Meadows, or the Precision Nutrition way that is simply using your hand to measure your protein, carbs, and fats.

I've heard countless people complain they can't lose the weight or get the health or body they want. However, after diving deeper with them, the majority of them are eating how they think is healthy or eating diet food.

They are frustrated!

But they don't know any better.

They thought just having a smoothie for breakfast and a salad for lunch would give them the results. It may help them make slow progress toward losing some weight, but it's not a high-performance style.

Maybe that's you.

Maybe you are frustrated because you feel stuck and you feel like you're not moving anywhere when you are eating the low-calorie foods, cutting out the sugar, cutting out fat, and eating less meat. These are usually the first things people go to first to make changes, but they are slow changes.

If you are tired of being frustrated, you need to fuel your body and get rid of the "lacking mentality" where you think you just need to cut everything out. Cut everything out and you'll end up craving and giving in. Then you'll go through that wicked and defeated cycle over and over again.

In combination with choosing the meal plan option that best fits your life and dialing into lifting weights, you will see faster results than just eating rabbit food or diet food and running blocks around the neighborhood or up and down the McKinley Monument.

As a high performer, you already have a lot on your plate. To make the nutrition part more doable, simplify it. Yes, there is the macro counting that professional competitors use, but do not be doubtful of the shape you can be in even without calculating every morsel that goes into your body. (If you do want extreme results, refer to prior chapters.)

To save time, you can hire a professional meal planning service to calculate and deliver your meals for you. But if you are doing it yourself, let's make it simple.

The simpler it is, the more likely you can do it without taking more energy away from the more important matters that require more time.

DO WHAT YOU BELIEVE IS BEST

People will be people.

Anyone and everyone has a voice these days, and it seems those who are the most popular and the loudest are heard. Being in the fitness and nutrition industry, even the professionals are at each other's throats for what they deem is right. It's hard to know where to start if these so-called professionals don't even agree.

I try to differentiate myself by understanding and respecting that everyone is different and unique. God made us that way. Whether you want to be vegan or not, what matters is getting in the protein first of all and balancing carbs and fats around it.

There are various styles to eat whether vegan, vegetarian, carnivore, paleo, keto, whole30, and many more. And there are pros and cons to almost anything out there. There is no perfect answer despite the loud egos trying to prove they are right. I want you to feel empowered to choose what is right and best for you. Then you can determine your customizable meal plan, while working with your doctor.

There are many healthy people groups around the world who eat very differently. It doesn't mean one group is right and the other is wrong—vegan, paleo, Indian, or Mexican. The best thing you can do is choose what you believe is healthy for you and your life.

What matters is you doing what you believe is healthy and taking steps in that direction. Choose what is best for you, your needs, your health, and your family.

There is still much to be discovered when it comes to nutrition. We've only hit the very tip of the iceberg on it, and I can honestly say I'm excited to continue learning as new discoveries come out.

For example, there's a great deal of supportive research and studies for the ketogenic diet, as well as against it. However, I personally work with Olympians who swear by the keto diet with intermittent fasting for their world-class results and testimonies and others who have lost over one hundred pounds and kept it off.

As long as it's okay with your doctor and it's something you can stick to while making your goals and becoming healthier, then do what's best for you.

"It's like bowling," Ciaran Fairman, PhD, stated as we met for coffee discussing nutrition and the wavering opinion of diet coaches available. "You have ten pins to knock down at the end of the lane. There's more than one way to do it."

Ciaran obtained his PhD in kinesiology and has published over fifty peer-reviewed abstracts, manuscripts, and book chapters in areas of exercise science and sports nutrition. We worked together in Major League Soccer and he continues to focus on the impact

of exercise, nutritional supplementation, and behavioral inter-
ventions on the health and wellness of those with cancer. So he
knows what he's talking about!

Your goal is get those pins down, and there really are many ways
to do it.

I personally purchase cage-free and grass-fed products, while
others call me selfish for eating meat at all. I feel good about it
because I buy from farmers I know are giving these animals a good
life. I'm supporting local farmers and a healthy life of the meat, so
they are raised with love and without additives. I don't buy from
stores anymore because it's hard to know the conditions of the
animals. I love supporting local farmers, but it's expensive. So to
meet my protein requirements for an athletic body, I drink protein
shakes and look for other protein sources.

If you don't like the sound of that at all and want to be vegetarian,
then be vegetarian. Want to be vegan? Then by all means, do it.
Don't make it complicated. Whichever you choose, you still need
enough protein whether you use plant-based options or meat.

If you have food sensitivities, as one out of three people do, then
simply remove those foods.

I can't have pork, eggs, dairy, peppers, most nuts, hemp, whey,
casein, beans, soy, and gluten. It's nearly impossible for me to have
a lean athletic body if I wanted to be vegan or vegetarian because
my body doesn't respond well to plant-based high protein.

Choose your version of healthy for you and your life, not somebody else's.

MAKE IT DOABLE FOR YOU AND YOUR LIFE

Whatever path you choose, I've found the way to get the best results is to have a high-protein diet, unless you decide you prefer keto. Most people who think they eat reasonably well and healthy discover they are eating only a small percentage of the protein they should be consuming.

Especially if dieting to get lean, people tend to eat less of everything, including the protein that is vital for making the physical changes they are aiming for. Remember those bowling pins?

Research shows that sedentary people need 0.3 grams of protein per pound of body weight, whereas athletes can use 1–1.1 grams. I'm an athlete and will die an athlete, so I aim for higher protein. Without it, I'm not eating like an athlete. Protein is part of my DNA and part of my purpose. With low amounts of it, I would not be a high performer.

You are what you eat, so eat quality food. Gut health is directly related to brain health and everything else. So for me, my nutrition goes beyond just being as fit and lean as I want to be, but because I want sources that contribute to a healthy microbiome. High performers need their minds, and they need clarity. I don't need another reason to seduce me to eating more doughnuts. I desire a healthy gut and what my body absorbs for ultimate function, not just for appearance and getting a better score on stage.

I try to rotate quality probiotics every few months according to Bob Wood, who is a pharmacist. "Our bodies need that stuff. Sometimes we are just buying dirt in a bottle, but it has all the strains necessary for a healthy gut, and it's best to introduce different kinds every three to four months for an optimal gut."

With an optimal gut, I can have optimal absorption, an optimal mind, and optimal performance. Fueling myself with high carbs, sugary or processed foods, chemicals, fast foods, and so forth isn't giving my body the fuel I am after to knock down all the pins. Instead, it slows it down with a bunch of gutter balls to go along with it.

CALCULATING

Most people think they have an idea of what they are eating and how much they are eating until they calculate it. I'm not suggesting doing this every day, but it's a great tool to see what and how much you really are consuming so you can adjust. It's fascinating to calculate occasionally to see if you really are eating what you think you are.

The majority of people think they have a good idea of what they are consuming, but after tracking, they realize how far off they are. Just because they are eating a salad every day for lunch and stop eating after 8:00 p.m. does not guarantee results. Let's just say, that's only a start!

When you think of the cream in your coffee, the leftovers your kid left behind, and pieces of candy here or there, it all adds up. Those little things still need to be considered. You may find out you are eating much less protein than you thought and more carbs, fats, and sugars. They sneak up on you if you aren't mindful.

To calculate, I prefer making it as simple as possible. Open a free account with myfitnesspal.com where you can plug in your current height, weight, sex, and your goals, whether you prefer to lose weight, stay the same, or gain weight. (Or if you have already used a formula from Chapter 5, then use those numbers.)

Once you have your total calories for the day, start adding in the foods you want to keep. Before I realized gluten was not a great thing for me, I used to calculate french toast with maple syrup and ate it every day. One of my clients, Billy, wanted a bacon, egg, and cheese breakfast muffin, so he calculated that in.

You already know you need around 1 gram of protein per pound of body weight (less if you are keto), so start adding proteins to get an idea of how much of that you need. After that, start calculating the carbs and fats.

To make it simple while still focusing on the more important things in life and being a high performer, don't calculate obsessively. Perhaps calculate just one time and make a point to eat all of that every day, rotating the foods so you don't get bored.

SIMPLIFY IN REAL LIFE

After years of competing, running my own business, and driving back and forth for my ill dad, I needed to find out how to simplify it all so I could focus on what matters more. If I didn't, it was too easy to forget meals, not get enough protein in, eat out, splurge on more breadsticks at Olive Garden and fast foods at drive-throughs.

The trick is setting yourself up for success. You do the same thing for your business and hopefully your marriage and family, which means you can do the same for your food. Don't let this worry you. I have mastered making this as simple as possible.

If you aren't having your healthy meals delivered to you or if you don't have your own personal chef, the following are ways to do it yourself.

MAKING MEALS EASIER AND HEALTHIER THAN EVER FOR OPTIMAL RESULTS

If you can't have meal prep service, then the simplest way is to have a list of your favorite and easiest high-protein recipes.

Most days, I just don't want to cook. I'd rather do anything else, but we need to eat. To make this as simple as possible, I have a list of my favorite high-protein recipes written on a dry erase board on my fridge.

There are many times I just don't want to cook (actually, it's like most of the time), but I can choose one simple recipe and have it ready in no time. Or for some recipes, I can throw simple ingredients into a Crock-Pot, knowing that dinner will be ready when we need to eat.

Easy high-protein and low-carb recipes (you can look these up online):

- Paleo stuffed peppers
- Gluten-free beer and onion soup mix roast beef (super easy in the Crock-Pot)
- Korean beef
- Paleo tacos
- Keto bacon blue-cheese burgers (this one is high in fat, so it's better with a low-carb diet)
- Lettuce wraps
- Zucchini boats (Italian style or taco style)
- Pork chops
- Zoodles with meat sauce
- Grilled steak
- Chicken chili

- Paleo chili without beans
- Peanut butter Buddha bowl
- Eggs and bacon with hot sauce Buddha bowl
- Shrimp on salad, gluten-free pasta, in a soup, as lettuce wraps, on kebabs
- Pulled pork
- Chicken and white bean soup
- Whole30 chicken shawarma
- Seiten (vegan)
- Paleo crispy chicken wings

Finding protein is the most important and first step of your customizable meal plan. After you have your protein, you can then add your vegetables, carbs, and fat.

In combination with many easy recipes, the combination of foods to enjoy is unlimited, especially when finding high-protein recipes that take little effort for the sake of being time efficient.

BATCH COOK SO YOU AREN'T COOKING FOR EVERY MEAL

Don't just make enough for one meal; make enough for a few days or even a whole week. Learn to be okay with leftovers or else you'll be wasting more time cooking than working on your high-performance life.

You are again setting yourself up for success, because even if you are busy, you can put some home-cooked food in a container, take it to the office, and grab a few protein shakes to go. There are benefits to having meals you can heat up and that are versatile, so you aren't eating the same thing every day.

For example, if you cook pulled pork, you can eat it plain one day; use a light BBQ sauce on it the next day; serve it with sauerkraut the third day; serve it with peach and mango salsa the fourth day; and eat paleo pork tacos on the fifth day. You have plenty of options to set yourself up for success.

Freeze half of it if you want to, then defrost it for a meal on another day.

MAKE IT EASIER FOR YOURSELF BY DETOXING PANTRY AND FRIDGE

Although I have worked incredibly hard for the discipline I have, if there are snacks somewhere in my house, I'm going to eat them unless I'm training for a competition.

Set yourself up for success by not having them around and snack on healthier options instead. If you do really want something anyway, go out and get yourself or your family a small serving of it.

I just can't buy a half-gallon of ice cream and think it'll just hang out there untouched. I will eat the whole darn thing. To set myself up for success, my family buys smaller portions. Or maybe I could have a little more discipline, but hey, not everyone is perfect. I'm just talking about setting yourself up for success, not tripping yourself up.

TAKE ALL YOUR FOOD WITH YOU

Carry a cooler with you if you need to. If you don't have the food with you, it's too easy to make a stop somewhere and throw a gutter ball. Gutter balls happen, but you don't want to make it a habit or you're just not going to have that great of a game. Bring the protein shakes and simple snacks to have with it like a thumb size of a fat like sunflower butter, raw almonds, or a small handful of fruit.

Worst-case scenario is, if you are traveling and cannot pack all of your meals, look at the menu in advance so you can make your healthiest selection when you order to keep succeeding. Ordering chicken, steak, or salmon salad with dressing on the side is my go-to. Many drive-throughs also offer grilled chicken sandwiches or burgers where you can ask for their low-carb version or without the bread. Some fast-food places will wrap it in lettuce for you to eat as a wrap, or you can eat it with a fork and knife.

MOST IMPORTANT MEALS OF THE DAY

Whether I'm training to be insanely lean or not, I'll still eat my slow carb, protein, and thumb-size portion of fat about an hour before working out. I'll consume great supplements before and during my training sessions, then I'll have fast carbs like white rice, protein, and a thumb-size portion of fat within sixty minutes. It's not complicated at all. Let the other meals fall around that.

By using these simple tips on nutrition, you'll be making progress because you are setting yourself up for success. Just don't make it more complicated than what it needs to be. I love how John Meadows stressed to his followers and athletes to not make this complicated.

If all else fails, try John's simple method.

- Breakfast: Eggs with spinach and vegetables, cooked in a half tablespoon of extra virgin coconut oil.

- Mid-Morning Snack: Chug a protein shake with a tablespoon of a nut butter or small handful of nuts.
- Lunch: Lean meat, size of your palm (double if a guy), thumb size of a fat like extra virgin olive oil for salad dressing on a bed of lettuce or drizzle over roasted vegetables. Cupped handful (two if a guy) of carbs like sweet potato. (Note: lean meat, such as chicken, turkey, lean beef, tuna, shrimp, or salmon. Fattier meat would be roast or pork, so you'd just eat a little less fat.)
- Afternoon Snack: Chug a protein shake with a tablespoon of a nut butter or small handful of nuts.
- Pre-Workout Meal: Something just like lunch. Using a slow-digesting carb like sweet potato or oats somewhere one to three hours before working out.
- Intra-Workout: Essential amino drink while lifting weights for about an hour.
- Post Workout: Dinner with family about forty-five minutes after training. This meal is just like your lunch, but eat a fast-absorbing carb like white rice, a bun, or pasta.

By using these tips along with a fine-tuned weight training program, you can simplify them both so you can become an overall higher performer. You are simplifying training and nutrition so you can still get in the best shape of your life in a much more balanced approach.

We've covered nutrition, so let's talk more about how beneficial weight training is to get the results you want. That's the topic of Part III!

KEY TAKEAWAY

The key is setting yourself up for success by making it simple. If you can pay to have someone calculate and deliver your meals, that's awesome. But aside from that, use the tips in this chapter and don't make it complicated.

Many times, I would be eating my meals as clients were getting dressed or undressed for their massage. It takes only two minutes. I don't need a twenty-minute break to chug a protein shake and eat a spoonful of almond butter.

HIGH-PERFORMANCE EXERCISE

Let's make this simple so you can set yourself up for success!

1. If I don't have the willpower or self-control over snacks (ice cream, cookies, chips, etc.) in my home, then I will donate them. True or false? Throw out or donate today.
2. Make a list of your favorite high-protein and low-carb recipes and batch cook.
3. Follow your customizable meal plan that you decided on either from Chapter 5 for extreme results or the Precision Nutrition method (measure with hand) in Chapter 6. Write out your customizable meal plan, and it's okay to tweak for best results.
4. Plan to lift weights for best results, timing carbs before and after training.
5. Regularly feed into your success and body and not starve it.

PART III

WEIGHTLIFTING

Right before starting my first massage appointment of the day, I ran into the restroom. I dropped my tights and underwear, only to notice the crotch of my panties weren't where they were supposed to be. It was on my hip and inside out.

How the heck was my underwear inside out and backward with the crotch on my hip?

I was in disbelief to how I got myself in this situation to begin with. Thankfully, nobody knew but me, but still, imagine wearing your underwear like that.

I had to run back to start my massage and probably wouldn't get a break later to correct my issue, so my crotch stayed on my hip all day.

All day.

So awkward and uncomfortable.

Stuff like that happens when you push yourself too far and with too much, with not enough time to recover. I was so exhausted trying to do my best at too much that I cracked eggs in my coffee instead of the skillet. Or I put cumin in my oatmeal instead of cinnamon which is absolutely disgusting. Or the day I backed my car out of the garage without opening the garage door.

You make stupid mistakes when pushing yourself beyond exhaustion. I know because I did it all the time. I had that no-pain, no-gain, no-rest mentality. I lived the life of seeing how much I could put on my plate, how much of my candle I could burn from both ends, and then I'd say yes to even more.

I was doing too much because I never dreamed of being average. Just know there are better ways than trying to conquer it all and spreading yourself too thin while lighting yourself on fire, then wondering where your crotch is.

There was a time, long, long ago, when if I wanted to lose weight and get in shape, I would mindlessly sweat on the treadmill and eat salads every day. I tried all the silly fad diets through my childhood, teen years, and even during my twenties to avoid the genetic obesity and diabetes that runs in my family.

I then paired the fad diets with sweat attacks on treadmills and cardio drills.

I did this until I learned a better way and sought out those who were already doing it.

I'm grateful I was in my snowboarding accident and had to learn how to walk again. I not only grew closer to God, but it opened the doors to taking my fitness career to a whole new level. A new hunger began. Not because I was dieting for competitions, but I was hungry to learn and grow.

I was hungry to take my forever growing mindset of a high performer, to focus on what matters most. It was more than just working harder, putting in extra hours, depriving your body, and running like a mad hamster on crack just for the sake of a sweat.

The best part is, if you are doing it right, you spend less time in the gym so you can focus on what matters most in life. You can have your mind clear so you remember to put your garage door up before you back out or can successfully wear your underwear.

Sometimes it's the little things, right?

TIME IN THE GYM

As a high performer, I am intentional about time management so I can be where it matters most. I want to be present with my husband, family, faith, and my work. There was a time where I thought just working out for the sake of working out was what made me a high performer, but that mindset didn't produce results.

I love what an Ironman told me about my training program:

> Between my older daughter starting high school, working long hours and training for a triathlon, I need to spend less time in the gym for strength training and bodybuilding. A three-day training workout fits perfectly into my current goals. Optimal training in less time will give me more time to swim, bike, and run, while being able to body build. A lot of people are very busy. They can fit this into their busy lifestyle.

Time is limited. Time is crucial. Time is something you don't want to waste.

You have people to love and dreams to pursue. You want more joy, confidence, and better health. You want the better body and you aren't going to waste or dwindle your time anymore.

Imagine the adventures. Imagine the dreams and goals. Imagine the deeper and more authentic relationships.

Imagine feeling joy in every area of your life. Imagine your finances taking leaps and bounds. Imagine being more productive. Imagine making time for travel, retreats, and your well-being.

Imagine crushing limits in your mind. Imagine how much more you could give back if you spent your time more efficiently. Imagine raising your kids in a healthy home. Imagine pouring into your faith that propels you even further.

This is the high-performance life.

CHAPTER 8

WHY I FELL IN LOVE WITH LIFTING AND WHY YOU SHOULD, TOO

Billy knows what matters most.

He's a husband, father of three, business owner, and hard worker, but he wasn't using time effectively to take care of his health. He was overweight and doctors were about to put him on high blood pressure medication.

I showed him my simplified version of weight training and nutrition, and he lost more than forty pounds in three months. He went to his next doctor's appointment and the doctor was shocked by the physical changes he had made and equally matched the changes internally.

He made such significant health improvements that he drastically lowered his blood pressure and learned how to do it by freeing time to be more present as husband and father of three so he could be present and perform even higher.

You can see him sharing the adoration and support of his wife and deepening faith, which plays a role in performing higher and doing what matters most.

Here is Billy's story, in his own words:

> I have an athletics background; I played almost every sport in high school and played semi-pro soccer after college. I probably fluctuated between 190 and 200 pounds out of high school. As my competitive career came to a close, I never learned what healthy eating and training meant, so I kept eating and drinking the same types and amounts of food I always had. So naturally, with the lack of nutrition and exercise, coupled with a family history of obesity, I slowly began to gain weight.
>
> I had people mention my weight to me, but for some reason, I never saw myself as overweight when I looked in the mirror. But I finally started coming to grips with it after I visited the doctor for a checkup. She told me that my weight was nearing 280 pounds and my blood pressure was high, so we may need to start looking at taking medication to get it under control. I knew I didn't want to take medication, but I didn't really know what to do.
>
> It wasn't until the fall of 2015 that something changed. I met Bailey when she and her husband, Andy, were visiting family in Memphis. I had known Andy from our time playing soccer and had kept in touch with him. Finding out that she had a background in fitness and coaching interested me, but I hadn't yet hit my rock bottom to have the desire to reach out and ask for help.
>
> Fast forward to February 2016. I was working from home for an online consulting company, married with a two-year-old and another baby expected in April. I had a wonderful life...or so it seemed.

In actuality, I was miserable at work. Even though I worked from home, I never left my desk and sat alone and isolated all day long. My weight had ballooned to near 300 pounds, and I wasn't doing anything for exercise. Basically, I had no social or physical outlets to work on my mental and physical health. I felt stuck in my walk with the Lord and did not have the motivation to go deeper. My wife knew it and had pleaded with me on a number of occasions to do something to get myself healthy.

One day, I got the news that my grandmother had passed away. She was about as close to me as my mom, and it rocked me. It wasn't too long after the funeral that my wife found me curled up in a ball crying my eyes out because of the state of depression I had found myself in. She cried with me and told me that she loved me and pleaded with me to make a change, not only for my health but the health of our family. She said, "Call Bailey and tell her where you are. Ask her if she will coach you. You need a coach to get started and have accountability. You have tried fads a million times and you always end up back to square one and frustrated. It's easier to steer a car in motion than one that is stuck in park.

So I called Bailey and shared everything. She listened and listened some more. She asked hard but important questions, and I remember her telling me that I needed to answer them out loud. I needed to state my fears and weaknesses. Then I needed to state my goals. I asked her, 'What if I don't know my goals?'

Bailey told me she would help me cultivate them, and she did. She set me up with a complete lifestyle shift. For three months, we had weekly video conferences, a strict eating plan, and a workout plan. It was enough time for me to break my unhealthy habits and develop some healthy ones. Enough time for me to listen, learn, engage, and take hold of my health.

All of this helped me learn that I don't have to stay in the unhealthy places that I was sitting in. I had freedom to make healthy changes. I felt freedom to quit my job, courage to say no to unhealthy lifestyle choices, and a will to say yes to JOY. I pursued things I was passionate about. I found more joy in being at home and with my family. I was able to speak my goals into existence. I hit plateaus like anyone, yet together we broke them down and pushed past them to continue moving toward my goals.

We started working together on Wednesday, March 23, 2016. I weighed in at 288 pounds and set a three-month goal to get to 255 pounds. By July 1, I weighed in at 247. I had lost more than forty pounds in just three months! Are you kidding me? Not only had the weight been coming off, but I went in for a physical with my doctor and she let me know that I had reduced my blood pressure to normal levels and would not need to take blood pressure medication. What an incredible win.

Bailey was an incredible blessing not just to me but to my entire family. She helped me recapture passions in me that I had forgotten I had. I followed the Lord's calling into working in ministry and rediscovered a passion for my marriage and family that I hadn't had in years. I continue to work out three to four times a week and maintain a healthy lifestyle. I owe an incredible amount of gratitude to Bailey for the wisdom, coaching, and heart she put into helping me achieve my goals.

THE IMPORTANCE OF WEIGHTLIFTING

It was meeting John Meadows that changed my way of thinking and the lies that I had to sweat every day. He took me under his wing to mentor me to winning my class in almost every show I've competed in, drawing diagrams explaining nutrition, and then he told me not to do too much cardio. I was stunned.

Everyone I knew who preached a healthy life did tons of cardio and spent more hours in the gym than I cared to.

But John was different. He said, "Too much cardio eats away at your muscle."

Muscle is what gives you shape, and you need to feed it to have the physique you want. Most people starve it and then go into hamster mode on wheels again and get slower and slower results.

It opened my eyes further to the physiques out there that were getting the results I was after. I wanted muscle, definition, and shape. I didn't want to be a slender "toned up" girl; that's just not me. I've always preferred reading muscle magazines for men for those workouts, not silly band exercises for butts mostly found in the women's magazines.

That just wasn't my thing.

Besides, men have the leanest and roundest glutes by doing all the basic movements, not the silly trendy workouts. There's a lot to be said for the basic movements.

I remember reading magazines to see how the models got to look like that. I would read their meal plans and the hours of work they put in every single week, and it just does not need to be that complicated.

The awesome thing about weight training is that it's a way to get the fastest results to the physique you want while saving time to do things that are even more important, like growing your mindset, business, well-being, relationships, and giving back to the community.

Lifting weights is more than just getting the body you want.

I fell in love with lifting weights because it was more than just the physical transformation that was happening faster than any other method, but it was because of finding who I was made of and what I was capable of. The feeling of getting stronger, being stretched mentally and physically. It's getting more in tune with your mind and body.

When I took it more seriously and competed on stage, the strength was beyond me, and I depended on my faith to eat and train at that level. The perk is that I did get the appearance that won trophies, titles, authority, and credibility.

Many people believe that weight training is only for the appearance of getting a great beach body, but what they don't know is the surprising health benefits for lifelong physical function, fitness, and performance. Maybe that's why I love it so much, because of the ability to have a lean and strong physique while achieving these powerfully healthy benefits.

And don't kid yourself. We all want to feel better in our own skin. We all want to feel sexy, whether you admit it or not. Especially if married, your spouse and your marriage is a gift, so treat it like that. Sex and desire is important to the health and performance of your marriage as well, so take care of yourself, for you and your marriage. There is nothing wrong with wanting to look good and feel good.

When you are taking better care of yourself with your health, longevity, and performance, you'll live a life full of vitality and vibrancy. The perk is that you feel and look better, too. More radiant, confident, stronger, leaner, and happier. Who wouldn't want that?

WHY WEIGHT TRAIN?

A recent study done at the University of Alabama at Birmingham compared dieters who just did cardio and dieters who just lifted three days a week. The results? Although they both lost the same amount of weight, it was those who lifted weights who lost more pure fat, while the cardio bunnies lost some valuable muscle and not just fat. With that being said, those lifting weights shed more body fat while adding definition to their bodies. (Hint, hint.)

If you are looking to make some changes, then weight training is where it's at.

You can:

- Lose body fat, earn a smaller waist, build a booty, gain muscle, or just get shredded
- Learn what successful physiques do to stay lean and strong
- Live the lifestyle and dream it takes to get your dream body, health, and confidence
- Develop the underlying qualities it takes that go beyond just the physical appearance

Let's look closer at these reasons why you are sexier when you lift weights.

ULTIMATE FAT BLASTER TO SHOW YOUR PHYSIQUE AND HARD WORK

Weight training is an ultimate fat blaster, especially when combined with a nutritious, high-protein diet. Those two combined right there will eat away fat much faster than cardio would. This is a no-brainer rule for the successful athletes and physiques out there.

Weight train three days a week to hit your major muscle groups for the most fat-burning results and feel like you don't need to live in the gym.

PURSUE DREAMS

Become stronger for a better quality of life and to pursue your dreams. If you are like most people and want to do great things before you die, then be committed to get strong now, build on it, and maintain it for decades to come. Turn that daydream into a reality! Watching people go for their dreams is pretty hot in my book.

Start with a personal trainer to guide you around the gym and show you how to use the equipment to prevent getting hurt. Watch trusted instructional videos. Visualize yourself executing a movement with perfect form before your workout, and make every rep better than the rep before. Don't just go through the motions. Activate the muscles you are isolating. This book will show you workout examples on exactly how to do that.

DISCOVER UNDERLYING QUALITIES

The number one reason why weight training is sexy is because muscle shows the underlying qualities it takes in a person to earn them beyond physical appearance. Sure, weight training is the secret ingredient to a faster metabolism and can make you visually appealing, but the people who are truly committed to it have deep soul-filled reasons why they love training with weights.

I conducted my own study, simply by asking people why they find men or women with muscle attractive. The results showed that they see more than just muscle, but they see inner strength that it takes to get there. They see confidence, self-respect, motivation, mental and physical growth, a positive mindset, character development, faith, discipline, maturity, and willpower. Everything sexy.

If you gain all of this while weight training, imagine the kind of energy in other areas of their life. #unstoppable

The awesome thing is that it doesn't have to be a dream or wishful thinking anymore. It can become a new lifestyle where you can learn how to lift weights only three days a week to burn the most fat, get the physique you want, and gain the strength, confidence, and sexiness.

THE SIX GREATEST BENEFITS OF LIFTING WEIGHTS

Whether you simply want to lose body fat, earn a smaller waist, build your booty, gain muscle mass, or just get shredded, the secret ingredient is lifting weights.

Still not convinced? Let's look at the seven biggest benefits you'll get from lifting weights.

BE A HIGHER PERFORMER

Save more time so you can be present at work and home, especially if you have a guided plan to training only three days a week.

BETTER MENTAL HEALTH

The mind and body are ultimately connected. Although your feelings can influence your movement or exercise, do you know that your workouts can influence your feelings anyway?

According to Harvard Medical School, studies have shown that regular exercise can improve mood disorders.[5] The way you move can affect the way you think and feel, so by moving more, you can also change your brain.

So when you aren't feeling like moving, convince yourself to get your workout in, whether it's dance, yoga, walking with a friend, martial arts, or lifting weights, for it all contributes to a healthier mind and body.

In fact, a study in twenty-four women who had been diagnosed with depression showed that exercise of any intensity significantly decreased feelings of depression.[6]

MORE CONFIDENCE MENTALLY AND PHYSICALLY

Confidence is not just a benefit of weight training; it's a war zone.

5   Srini Pillay, "How Simply Moving Benefits Your Mental Health," *Harvard Health Blog*, Harvard Health Publishing, Mach 28, 2016, https://www.health.harvard.edu/blog/how-simply-moving-benefits-your-mental-health-201603289350.

6   Jacob D. Meyer et al., "Influence of Exercise Intensity for Improving Depressed Mood in Depression: A Dose-Response Study," *Behavior Therapy* 47, no. 4 (July 2016): 527–537, https://doi.org/10.1016/j.beth.2016.04.003.

Confidence is something to fight for and believe in because there are so many things that would try to make you believe otherwise.

Confidence is one important attribute I want for everyone; however, it isn't something I can give. I can encourage someone until I am blue in the face, but ultimately it is up to them to believe it.

Confidence is something for you to fight for, to believe in, to live out, to pass along to those around you. Confidence is to build yourself and others around you, to give your best, and believe your best. Confidence is loving yourself and your progress in every stage of life. Confidence is sexy and the sexiest thing you could be.

Not to mention the extra confidence having a solid plan where you can save time and put toward what matters most.

STRONGER BONES AND JOINTS (WHICH MEANS FEWER INJURIES)

Whereas it's easier to have stronger bones and joints while young, those characteristics are easily taken for granted, since they break down as we age.

Later in life, new bone tissue doesn't get created as quickly. This is especially pronounced among people who are sedentary and women who have reached or passed menopause. The bone tissue loss leads to the weakness and postural problems that plague many older adults.

"To me, resistance training is the most important form of training for overall health and wellness," says Brad Schoenfeld, an assistant professor of exercise science at New York City's Lehman College.

Interviewed by *Time* magazine, he added, "Resistance training counteracts all those bone losses and postural deficits."[7]

Through a process known as bone remodeling, strength training stimulates the development of bone osteoblasts, cells that build bones back up. Although you can achieve some of these bone benefits through aerobic exercise, especially in your lower body, resistance training is really the best way to maintain and enhance total-body bone strength.

BURN MORE BODY FAT

Lifting weights not only burns more calories for hours after training, but when building lean muscle, the fat comes off even faster. Muscle is a big fat burner. Of course, nutrition plays a huge role in this as well, but when it comes to exercises and movement, weight training can streamline your fat loss.

Fat burning happens faster with weight training than with any kind of cardio exercise. Although cardio has many health benefits in itself, the point here is that muscle burns fat faster than cardio.

When you lift weights while using proper nutrition, you can gain more muscle. When gaining muscle, it creates a burning stove within your body that burns calories and fat, while building shape.

GET A GREAT PHYSIQUE

The physiques that are winning competitions aren't doing crazy

---

7   Markham Heid, "Why Weight Training Is Ridiculously Good for You," *Time*, June 6, 2017, https://time.com/4803697/bodybuilding-strength-training/.

cardio sessions and eating salads all day. They are lifting weights and eating higher amounts of protein.

Of course, there is cardio mingled in, but the base of a great-shaped body comes from resistance training with weights, bands, or body weight. In fact, by doing too much cardio, not only will you be burning fat, but you'll be burning away your muscle, too.

DISEASE PREVENTION

Weight training is a great way to prevent and battle obesity to decrease your risk of diseases and health problems, such as heart disease, diabetes, and high blood pressure.

INCREASING IMMUNITY

COVID-19 opened my eyes to this one. In our lifetime, it has never been more important to be more focused on increasing overall immunity. We get sick. We all do. Weightlifting along with increasing overall metabolic health increases your ability to recover. Read more in *The Immunity Fix* by Dr. James DiNicolantonio and biohacking coach Siim Land.

LIFTING WEIGHTS THREE DAYS A WEEK FOR MAXIMUM RESULTS IN MINIMAL TIME

The goal of this book is to help you achieve overall success. I want you to get more done in half the time, and I'm guessing you would like more time to put toward the more important things in your life as well.

By focusing on the largest muscle groups while lifting weights only three days a week, you'll get yourself the results you are after at a much faster rate.

I mean, if you prefer working out six days a week and would rather not save yourself some time in the gym to put it toward the more important things in your life, then that's okay. Many look at gym time as therapy time, mental health time, or sanctuary time.

Because you are a high performer, you are strategic with your time; you know that it's crucial and sacred to you. You invest into your time; you don't throw it around and hope for the best. You make plans to do what it takes to become your best.

According to Brendon Burchard's research, the top 5 percent of the highest performers work out three days a week. If you are even in a smaller niche of that 5 percent and want to have the body of your dreams in minimal time so you can perform even higher in all areas of your life, then this is how you can do it successfully.

Each week, find where you can get into the gym and train for one hour per day, three days a week.

The simplest breakdown is to train three days a week, every week, for one hour.

- Day One: Back and Biceps
- Day Two: Chest, Shoulders, and Triceps
- Day Three: Legs and Glutes
- Day Four (optional): Add a fourth training day for a lagging body part if you'd like and the rest of your life permits it.

Sure, you can move these around, but this is the simplest breakdown. Let's say you want one day for just training arms and shoulders. That's fine; train them as your fourth training day.

Give yourself one simple rule when it comes to lifting weights: just get all three done by the end of the week. Nothing more complicated than that. Just get those three days in.

If you have to travel or have plans, do your best to squeeze those workouts in before you leave. Sure, there are body weight and band exercises that you can do while traveling, but it doesn't get the maximum results as if using dumbbells, bars, plates, and cables. You'll still get results but not maximum results in minimal time.

This is how to get maximum results in minimal time so you can still perform higher in all the other areas of your life, while being present and happy at the same time.

If you don't want maximum results, it's okay. You don't have to lift weights, but that's how you get the results deep down you really want. If not, you'll have to spend more time doing the other modes of working out, taking valuable time away where it matters most.

If you want a High Performance life while getting in the best shape you've ever been in, this is exactly how you do it. Now, if you want to hike, swim, and dance, then by all means, go do what you enjoy. Just know if you want maximum results with your body in minimal time, you get those results by lifting weights and following this chapter. If you want the other activities, use them as your active rest days, so your priority is lifting but other days can have activities you enjoy.

For example, in the winter I am a snowboard instructor and competitor. I purposely train legs and glutes one or two days prior to snowboarding. I use the snowboarding not only for fun but to shake out the soreness from training. You can do the same with spin class, yoga, hiking, Zumba, kickboxing, or martial arts. You can still do what you enjoy.

I know when I was competing against women using steroids, when I wasn't even using fat burners, I needed to have larger and more rounded shoulders to even stand a chance. I made my fourth training day just for shoulders while following my meal plan, and finishing in the top ten on an NPC national stage, all without the drugs or fat burners. I did it all while owning and running my business, date nights with my husband, and traveling to help my family with my dad who was diagnosed with ALS. It was while keeping the important things a priority.

To really make the most of this way of training, I'll get into advanced techniques, such as breathing and mind-muscle connection. I love it because I've adapted it from building muscle, conditioning, and lean body fat percentage in competitions in minimal time. It helps to maximize your results, too.

If you are the type of person who wants to look like they could compete but without actually doing a show, this is for you, too. You can even use this as a foundation for contest prep with a few tweaks if you want. However, even those who don't want to actually step on stage, want to have the physique and fitness level as if they potentially could. This is your ticket to getting there.

HIIT WORKOUTS

It may take a week or two to get yourself trained to prioritizing weightlifting and its intensity. After that, add a day of high-intensity interval training, HIIT, for twenty to forty-five minutes of what you like, just not slow and steady.

Once you've gotten the rhythm of training three days a week and then your one day of HIIT, add your second day of HIIT. I prefer to do my HIIT after training back and training chest. If I'm a little behind or run out of time, I'll do HIIT on its own day at the gym or sometimes outside. The great thing is that you can make this work for your life.

Although most people think they need to bust their ass on a treadmill or StairMaster and then add in some weights or hire a trainer later, you'll get somewhere faster by switching those priorities around.

Lift weights as number one and HIIT as number two. The weights are your fundamentals. It's your base. It's your strength. It's where you create the definition and shape you really want.

HIIT helps to shed extra body fat and increase metabolic health to show the definition and shape you've worked hard for. So if you are planning for an event where you want to be in your best shape, train three days a week, add a fourth for a lagging body part if you really want, and then increase the intensity and frequency of HIIT leading up to your event.

Usually when people want to lose body fat and get healthy, they tend to become cardio bunnies and eat like bunnies. Cardio is not the first thing to go to if you want fast and amazing results. If you notice people who are obsessed with cardio versus people who are obsessed with weight training, you'll see the people lifting weights (if doing it correctly) have more shape and are more lean and stronger than the ones just trying to get a good sweat doing cardio.

Seriously, the magic happens with lifting weights, HIIT, and fueling your body properly.

With cardio, to get extreme results in minimal time, it isn't long and steady cardio but instead HIIT. I keep mine super simple and walk on an incline on a treadmill, spin class, or get on a StairMaster. Nothing complicated or time consuming at all.

Seriously. Keep this simple as it should be. Don't overthink it.

If I had convenient stairs around me, I'd prefer to do them outdoors. Don't make it more complicated, but look up HIIT workouts, and do them after lifting weights or on off days up to two to three days a week.

I find cardio to be best after lifting so your energy is going into pushing weights for ultimate transformation, and not getting the energy that is left over. If you do best doing cardio before, then do what works best for you.

Instead of long and steady cardio, you only need a good twenty to forty-five minutes of HIIT either after you train back or chest or do it on off days. John Meadows prefers not doing cardio or HIIT after training legs, so I listen to the legend himself.

Remember, listen to the ones who do it successfully.

After that, squeeze a few rounds of ab workouts either at the end of training, or you can do it between sets to save even more time, depending on your preference. That may take only ten minutes a week, sometimes less. You are already training your core when doing bench, squats, and dead lifts.

You don't need an entire day just for abs.

It has been quite freeing and enlightening to get in the best shape of my life. I can maximize my time in the gym to get maximum results, while performing higher in other areas of my life as well. We don't have a zillion hours in a day; we have only twenty-four, so it makes me have a better relationship with time to perform even higher.

Now that you know how great this is for your health, let me show you how to get faster results in less time so you can still perform high in all areas.

KEY TAKEAWAY

Lifting weights is much more than just looking good. It goes much deeper than that. From mental health, bone health, stronger immune system, and more confidence, to simply getting the fastest results possible to being in the best shape of your life. If you are a high performer wanting to perform higher in every area of your life without living in the gym and without obsessing over calories and macros, then this is your guide to the overall higher performing life while getting maximum results in minimal time.

HIGH-PERFORMANCE EXERCISE

1. Before you start your day, continue to visualize where you want to go, what you want to feel, where you want to be, what your family and marriage looks like/feels like, and so forth.

2. Pick your three days for weightlifting. Schedule one hour for each of those three days. If you can't do an hour just yet, start with thirty minutes. Instead of three days where you'll get the best results, try four or five days of thirty to forty-five minutes until you can work toward one hour.

3. Continue to fuel your gut, body, muscle, mind, and workouts with quality nutrition and supplements. You are what you absorb.

CHAPTER 9

HOW TO GET FASTER RESULTS WITH WEIGHT TRAINING AND YOUR HIGH-PERFORMANCE LIFE

My dad always told me, "Whatever you do, do it with everything you have."

Even as a teenage drive-through girl for McDonald's, I gave my best, even if it wasn't what I felt like. I had a big smile on my face, chose eye contact with each customer who was usually grumpy and demanding, and wanted to give their experience my best, too.

McDonald's coffee cups have a line to show how high we were supposed to fill them with hot coffee. Customers would be angry that I "only" filled their cups to the line and thought I was ripping them off by not filling it to the top. But if I had filled it above the line to avoid their grumpy pants, more would complain that I was trying to burn them! Most people arrived at the window grumpy, taking their day out on me. But I had to do my best to work with everything I had, including my attitude.

In college, I worked in sales. At first, I didn't even know what I'd been hired for; I only knew the scripts. I helped people schedule times for someone to go to their house and preplan their wishes and cemetery plots so it wouldn't leave a burden on the family when they die. Someone on the other end of the phone once called me the grim reaper!

Later, I was a demonstration model for Godiva Chocolate. I had to serve chocolates on a crystal plate held over my head as if I were some fancy lady in a black dress. Anytime I had to go to the back room to fill up the plate, I probably put more in my mouth instead of on the plate and was sick for days. But I did my best!

Whether I was throwing a baseball, hurdling for the track team, running my own business, or hating my fast-food job, I've always done my best.

It's in the Bible, too.

"Whatever you do, work at it with all your heart." Colossians 3:24

"Above all else, guard your heart, for everything you do flows from it." Proverbs 4:23

Do it with your whole heart, and guard it.

It's sacred.

This mindset spilled over into every other area of my life. Whether I wanted to give every person I touched the best massage they have ever had or to listen to my coaches with everything I had to give my best, serving the community, or doing random acts of kindness where nobody would ever know it was me, I gave my best.

It's part of developing character and integrity, not for the sake of being seen.

Even with time that we are given, I wanted to give my very best. Not just when I'm being seen on stage, but the biggest transformations take place when nobody is watching. It's a mindset to create a habit to take everywhere with you.

When I get to the end of my day, I ask myself if I did what mattered most in the hours and moments I had. At the beginning of my day, I ask myself what matters most and whatever it takes to do that.

FEEL IT

This mindset is even poured into my training style. If we have only seven days a week and twenty-four hours a day, by the time you map out your days for work, training, marriage, family, and time for renewing your mind and body, not much time is left over, so what matters is being present and intentional in all of it.

You need to feel it.

So many people go through life unsure of meaning and purpose, causing doubt and depression, yet they fear feeling things. They want to get through life on knowledge and pure effort; however, that's only a small part of the equation.

It's okay to feel things and to pray how to respond. Without it, you begin to lose sense of purpose.

At the end of the day when I ask myself if I did what matters most today, I'll go back and reflect on that moment and feel it. I intentionally take myself back to the moment and feel the feels I did when I first experienced it. Whether the tears welling up in my eyes as clients experience breakthrough or the look of pure joy and excitement as my toddler lit up seeing her birthday cake with candles.

High performers do not go through life checking off lists and simply becoming rich. Or just to do it all over the next day. That begins to feed into a mindset where you forget to feel and you lose your purpose and meaning to what matters most in life. You can't have it without feeling it.

If you struggle with feeling, don't hesitate to work with counselors and coaches to teach you and guide you. I love mine and without them, I probably would be another person checking off tasks and wandering around without a greater purpose. Feelings are good; just don't let them direct your life.

Do what you need to do to feel healthy physically, emotionally, mentally, and spiritually.

In my premarital classes, we talked about healthy emotions and how emotions are like a smoke alarm. It could be an alarm showing you where the smoke is and where the fire is. Some try to take the batteries out of the smoke alarm because they don't want to hear it, but meanwhile, everything burns down.

Give and get the most out of your time, and make it work for you. Don't waste it. When you do, you live more with purpose and meaning and get faster results. You aren't wandering anymore without direction and intention.

The mindset applies to training and nutrition to get the fastest results like Billy did in Chapter 8. It's not about just showing up and doing three sets of this exercise and three sets of that or how many rounds you can do for time, but it includes intentionality for every single repetition to give it your best.

Weight training does give the fastest results but with very mindful reps and intentional nutrition. Maybe you've experienced this, where you grab some weights and work really hard, sweating your butt off, but not really feeling or seeing much of a difference.

When you apply your energy into weight training, that's where the magic is. If you spin it all out in the hamster wheel, you won't have much space left for a workout with impeccable form.

When you use impeccable form, you create a stronger mind-muscle connection that not only protects you from injury, but you intentionally drive all of your mental energy through making that movement. Focus on making every single rep even better than the rep before, which gets harder and harder, but that's where the magic is...not the wheel.

Just as you need to feel life, feel purpose, live with your heart, and guard your heart, you need to feel every single repetition. You give your best. Give your all. Give your heart and feel it.

Focus on making each rep even more perfect than the rep before or else you'll find yourself sloppy and using time ineffectively. When you make each rep as best as you can as the one before it, you are engaging more of your muscle, more of your mind, and more of your energy.

Some sloppily sling weights around, but in order to get the physique that they want, they will have to do many more reps and more training days than you. So the key to having fewer training days so you can grow everywhere else is having impeccable form while using challenging weight.

MIND-MUSCLE CONNECTION

I love the feeling of being in the zone when I walk into the gym. I've already looked at my workout in advance, knowing exactly what I'm about to do. This time is completely dedicated to training, not answering calls, emails, or checking notifications.

I already ate my pre-workout meal about an hour prior, and I'm ready to get the most out of every single repetition for the next hour. Earbuds are in. I have my essential amino acids in my shaker cup that I am already sipping on. It's go-time.

Wherever you are, be all there, especially at the gym.

To make that mind-muscle connection, it's more than just seeing how much weight you can bench. It is reminding yourself the most important tasks to execute the movement like the arch in your back, feet on the ground, the power of your breath pushing the bar up, and if you are using a narrow, mid-grip, or wide grip on the bar.

It is visualizing in your mind exactly how it feels to bench. You reflect back to your best moments benching. Whether it was the way you arched your back, the way you engaged your lats as you pushed up the bar, or the explosive strength pushing the bar up, go back to that moment.

You remember how it felt. Your muscles remember how it felt.

Mentally connect to what that felt like physically within your body and mind.

You'll get tired, but if you don't keep yourself in check, your form will get sloppy, and then you are prone to injury and you won't get the most out of your workout. This is why you want to make every repetition better than the rep before. Because you will get tired and exhausted and will need to mentally coach yourself, "Arch the back, feet down, squeeze the lats, exhale on the push up." When I am getting really exhausted and don't think I have any more good reps in me, I focus on my attention in my feet. Focus on pressing your feet hard into the floor and you'll find another blast of energy.

Close your eyes if you have to to feel it before you even lift off the bar. One task I challenge myself with is relaxing my lips and jaw when I am pushing my limits. Or relaxing the upper traps while engaging lats since most people have the tendency to overactivate their traps.

Don't just use this for the bench press, but use it for every exercise, just as you have been doing your life wheel and one year from now every morning.

HOW TO GET FASTER RESULTS

Here are some quick tips to get faster results from your training:

- Focus three days a week on concentrated workouts.
- Minimal cardio after training back or chest, or even on an off day or two if you prefer.

- Sprinkle ab and calf exercises in once or twice a week after workouts.
- Add a fourth training day for a lagging body part, but don't forget the importance of being an overall higher performer, not just in the gym.
- Focus on perfecting your form even more so when you are tired. Don't ever get sloppy.
- Use warm-up sets to really prime your muscles and joints well. Once you are warmed up and can add more challenging weights, that's when you should start counting unless you are a beginner, and then that could be too much. See more in Chapter 10 for how to adjust this to your level.

KEY TAKEAWAY

Do you ever see those unbelievable transformation stories that make your eyeballs pop out of your head, wishing that could be you? Those transformations actually happen more often than you realize and it doesn't need to be complicated. It happens with lifting weights as the magic maker and dialing in your nutrition.

I watched so many competitors lose their marriage, sanity, and family because they thought they had to work out two to three hours a day, multiple days a week. I was winning most of the competitions lifting weights only three to four days a week with minimal cardio, plus I kept my sanity. I'm not saying that to brag, but I'm saying that to shed light on the fact it doesn't need to be as complicated as people make it out to be.

When people want to start getting healthier, lose body fat, or get ready for a big day, they usually blast time on a treadmill or elliptical, but that is the LAST place you'll find results. Sure, it's better than doing nothing, but high performers don't just blast away without a strategy in their business or in the gym. This is one of the ways they achieve a High Performance lifestyle and sustain it, and so can you.

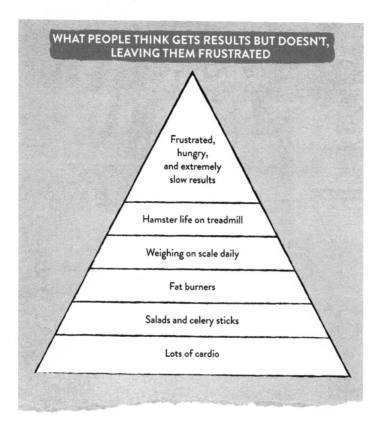

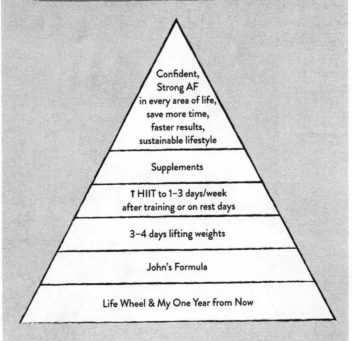

HOW TO GET MAX RESULTS AND KICK ASS IN LIFE

Confident,
Strong AF
in every area of life,
save more time,
faster results,
sustainable lifestyle

Supplements

↑ HIIT to 1–3 days/week
after training or on rest days

3–4 days lifting weights

John's Formula

Life Wheel & My One Year from Now

HIGH-PERFORMANCE EXERCISE

Focus on those three days per week and make a simple rule with yourself to make sure you get those three by the end of the week. Watch and feel for your transformation when paired with dialed-in nutrition. Abs and calves just do once a week, and save cardio for your leftover energy after training or off days.

When you give and get the most of your time in the gym, you'll be able to see faster results, plus save time you can't ever get back. Time you can spend on business, travel, family, retreats, self-care, community service, and hobbies.

Now that you have the foundation for getting the best results between nutrition and weights, you can fine-tune the dial in your workouts for exactly where you are and how far you want to go.

1. When you wake up in the morning, visualize and feel the feels of where you will be in one year from now by focusing on the High Performance life and making *Three Days Strong AF* your lifestyle.
2. Whatever matters most, *do that.* On your agenda for the day, think of the moments that may matter most. Imagine the people you are connecting with, whether employees, family, spouse, clients, and so on. The barista. How do you want them to feel? Visualize your day with your workout, your nutrition, a meeting with a client, a phone call, finish writing a strategy, going to an event, or flying a kite with your kid. Visualize what matters most every morning.
3. At the end of the day, reflect back on those moments. Relive them. How do you feel about them? Need to work on connecting a little more? Being better on time management? Feel good for your workout? If not, do you need better nutrition somewhere? Did you give your workout 100 percent? The moments you feel grateful for? The moments you feel like you need a lot of work? Give it to God and practice this routine each day for self-mastery.

CHAPTER 10

HOW TO DIAL IN YOUR INTENSITY FROM BEGINNERS TO THE ELITE

I had dreams of being a pregnant lady who still lifted weights and ate healthy. I was going to be a badass through my pregnancy. I had this disciplined lifestyle down to a science. I made it a habit every day, and I wasn't going to blink when it came time to grow a baby. I was excited to continue bench pressing, squatting, deadlifting, and just maintaining my strength. Nothing super heavy but enough to stay active, strong, and nothing more than what I was already doing.

And then, once that miracle was in there, I learned that discipline had nothing to do with it.

I was so sick through the entire pregnancy. I couldn't think of anything but Coke to eat or drink that wouldn't come back up.

It wasn't just the first trimester, when they say the morning sickness is supposed to subside; it was all day and through the entire pregnancy. I felt like I had the flu for nine months. The thought of food, water, or even brushing my teeth made me throw up for nine months. (In fact, it wasn't until after the baby was born was I able to not throw up at the thought of food and water, and brushing my teeth still makes me gag now.)

My dreams of being a badass pregnant lady were gone.

I was on injections and medication for the last four months to keep the baby in there due to preterm labor, and I was informed to not lift. I had an emergency C-section, which is a major surgery, and had to wait three months for proper healing. I had and still struggle with hernia and diastasis recti where my abs are split apart 4 cm and I look pregnant if you'd catch me relaxing from the side view. It's not a beer gut; my ab walls are just torn apart.

Finally, I was happy to be cleared to get into the gym again. The first week, I realized how much physical strength I had lost and how much mental strength I was ready to gain.

I couldn't do simple squats. I removed all the plates from the squat bar and still felt unsafe just moving the bar by itself. Man, I'd lost more strength than I ever thought possible.

Humbling, but I stood in front of the mirror without any weight at all and just focused on lowering my body into a squat position and learning to fire my glutes again. I got down on my knees to do push-ups, and found I could do only five, and that was with taking breaks and my arms shaking.

I had to learn to adjust the dial of my intensity. I wasn't where I was before I was pregnant and it was time to start over.

What if people were watching? What if they laughed at me?

I told myself, "You know what? Every single person has as much right to be in the gym working on their health and fitness as the next. Whether overweight and self-conscious, not knowing how to do anything or where to start, afraid of people looking at you, insecure about your body, or gym etiquette, we all start somewhere. You have grace and patience for others in the gym; it's time you have some for yourself, too."

USE YOUR DIAL

Have laser focus for your goals when you are in the gym. Whether you are just starting out or you're a professional athlete and everyone in between; each person has a dial.

If I had continued my tough intensity through my pregnancy, it may have not turned out so well. I had to adjust. If I cranked that dial up to a ten immediately following my C-section, that would not have been wise, so I lowered my dial and my intensity level.

When using *Three Days Strong AF*, you will learn how to adjust your training intensity to prevent injury and get the best results possible for your level.

My client Jared learned to adjust his dial when he started working out after being away from the gym for a while. He was so excited to get started on training three days a week so he could still work full time, serve his church as a musician, and have time to meet his future wife. Jared really wanted to lose weight, get strong and lean, and improve his overall health.

Because he hadn't been active in a long time, I advised him to take it easy getting started. It's important to know what level you are and ease into it.

The next few days, I wasn't surprised to hear how sore Jared was. He was so excited to get his results that he went full throttle as if he had been lifting for years.

"I can barely move and I think I injured my shoulder, so I'll need to take a few weeks off," he told me.

Don't be like Jared! He was so excited to start this program that it took him two weeks to heal to stay on the journey. There is nothing to be gained when you are injured like that, except time off.

Beginners (or people who haven't lifted in months) need to think about how much they can lift and then maybe lift only 60 percent of that. You may not even feel it while doing it, but you'll be in so much pain the next two days or even longer that it's harder to get back to the gym. Remember, set yourself up for success.

Ease into it. Once you get adjusted, then slowly increase the weight. As you advance and adjust, you can challenge yourself even more by adding chains and bands in addition to the weight. I find it better to lift less in your first week starting so you can reevaluate. From there, you can decide if you need more or not without injuring yourself or setting yourself back.

Perhaps you already have this mastered. Perhaps you already train three days a week or more in the gym, while advancing your career, improving your health, and relationships. Maybe you know to adjust your dial and intensity, know when to rest, and know how to keep your marriage, faith, and family a priority. You focus on performing well and advancing your career or projects. You over-come hiccups in life and adjust accordingly instead of allowing the stresses in life to knock the feet from under you. You practice healthy habits to keep it all balanced while moving forward.

If so, great! You are on the right track. But you can always get better, no matter what level you're at.

Your limits begin and end in your mind. So if you want lasting change in your mind and body, you can achieve it. Wherever you are, you can make improvements relationally, physically, spiritually, emotionally, or financially and with your weight training.

Let's look at some different training techniques and tips for begin-ners, intermediate, and advanced high performers.

BEGINNING TRAINING LEVEL

If it's been a while since lifting, this is a great place to start. You don't want to be starting off advanced or driving yourself into the ground with the dial blasted at a ten because that's where you can really hurt yourself, like Jared did.

I know you are excited, but be smart and patient with yourself. Ease into it; loosen up your joints; use perfect form, stretch, and teach those muscles of yours to activate. You'll experience sore-ness, but be smart.

Even when I came back to the gym after my emergency C-section, I adjusted my own dial from where I used to be to where I really needed to be for the sake of safety. I lowered my intensity and started lifting like a beginner again and was totally okay with that.

Humbling, too, but we all need to be humbled sometimes.

If starting off as a beginner, instead of lifting 100 percent, maybe drop that intensity down to 60 percent of what you think you really are capable of, and maybe even a little less. Focus on getting the three days in every week, and then eventually increase the weight, and wait a few weeks before adding cardio.

By waiting to add cardio, you begin building your new lifestyle habit of making weight training the priority.

It gives your mind and muscle time to train to activate the right muscles, learn how to breathe, learn how to rest between sets, and use perfect form. If you go too heavy and too intense in the beginning, you are risking injury, bad form, and being too sore to come back and stay on schedule.

I typically have two or three warm-up sets of exercises before I even start counting the sets on a more advanced level. This helps to warm up the joints and activate the correct muscle. Doing this is awesome, but if you are brand new or coming back after a long time off like I did, including all the warm-up sets is just too much.

Dialing down my intensity and starting safely as a beginner made me remove some of the sets instead of including the two to three warm-up sets plus three or more actual working sets. There are usually four or more exercises to follow, and it was just too much for me when starting off.

I only did warm-up sets to get things moving my first week or two. When I started to feel a little stronger, I was able to add another set, or go from 60 percent weight to 65 percent weight.

If you're a beginner, there's no need to use heavy weight yet, but instead focus on form and just getting in your three workouts every week. No need to kill it or get crazy. It's to focus on making this a lifestyle and you can control your own dial.

Ease into it and be smart. As you adapt, challenge yourself a little more. Challenge yourself; don't hurt yourself.

You may be able to do only a few sets of each exercise and that's okay. Everyone starts somewhere. Don't set yourself back by being too intense too early and hurting yourself.

INTERMEDIATE TRAINING LEVEL

At an intermediate level, you can start increasing weight a little bit. If as a beginner you've gotten yourself up to 65 percent or 70 percent, maybe you can go up a little bit more—perhaps to 75 percent—as long as you are still being challenged.

Just make sure you are using perfect form, activating the right muscles, all while challenging your strength, or you'll just be another guy in the gym throwing weights around. Every single movement should have a purpose.

Keep practicing and every single rep is an opportunity to make it a better one. Just get in your three days every week.

Watch training videos before getting to the gym to visualize in your mind exactly what you are going to do at the gym.

Start getting into your own head. Don't wait for a coach or trainer to be in your face telling you what to do, but take responsibility and become your own coach in your own mind. I've known many people to hire trainers, but they stay at the same place. It's up to you to become one in your mind for the sake of your own discipline and success.

Talk yourself through it. Wear earbuds and listen to music to block everything out so your small window of time gets all of your attention. There are times I lie down on the bench with my earbuds blocking out distraction and in my mind pumping myself up, saying, "You got this. Grip here, get your feet on the floor, get that arch in your lower back, watch your wrists, breathe in when lowering the weight, hold the barbell on my chest and hold your breath for a second, and drive up and exhale pushing the weight up. 3, 2, 1, GO!"

You don't want to sloppily go through the motions for the sake of just getting it done, or you won't be activating muscles, getting stronger, or seeing results. Anything you do in life takes intentionality.

You should be doing all your warm-up sets and working sets.

Feel yourself being challenged but in a healthy way, making every single repetition better than the one before.

Can you really make the rep better than the rep before? Maybe not, but in your mind, it keeps you from getting lazy on form. It's nice because when you are close to exhaustion in the middle of a set, if you focus on your breath and your form, you'll dig deeper to explode the weight.

For example, when bench pressing, it's easy for the chest to start exhausting. Mentally put your focus from your chest, into your heels driving through the ground or your lats assisting your pecs to execute the movement. You'll find more strength, even when you thought you were done.

Once training three days a week is a habit and a priority, then add cardio and abs after training chest or back, but not after legs. Either that, or do cardio and abs on off days.

Training first allows you to pour your energy into where it matters most; that way, cardio gets whatever energy you have left.

Nobody is the same, so I've worked with a professional competitor and IFBB Pro who only knew how to do cardio first and didn't know how to change and preferred it that way. Do what works for you. Lots of energy is still getting to the weight training where all the magic happens, so that's what matters most.

Doing only cardio and no weights can help lose body fat, but doesn't give you the extreme results or shape most people are after. Remember, the most impressive physiques lift weights; they're not running in hamster wheels, so it depends on what you want to do. This is my proven guide to help you become a high performer while getting strong and lean in minimal time, and the magic is in lifting weights, not cardio.

Run if you want to be a runner. Run if you enjoy it. However, if you are after results, then run after doing your workouts.

ADVANCED TRAINING LEVEL

If you have been training for a while, you are your own coach in your mind and even stronger than before. You are giving 100 percent with all of your warm-up sets, activating and isolating the muscle you are working.

To take it to the next level, you are not only controlling your breathing but owning mind-muscle activation in controlled movements.

You are counting the seconds of your rest time between sets like a hawk to not waste any time or letting your muscles get cold.

You can add bands to add assistance or resistance to your squats, dead lifts, and bench press. You can add chains to the same exercises to stimulate muscle activation, growth, and greater challenge. That feeling of max explosion is delicious.

Yes, I said delicious.

You are using supplements to give you the results you want during your workout while your glycogen transporters are allowing glycogen to refuel and feed your muscles. I consider this the most important meal of the day.

If you prefer a higher heart rate, you can work on abs during rest time as long as it isn't taking energy away from your lifts.

Challenge yourself with your mind-muscle connection while lifting. You aren't just throwing weights; every single movement is intentional.

TRAINING MORE THAN THREE DAYS A WEEK AND THE IMPORTANCE OF RECOVERY

You can train more than three days a week if you want, but don't let the fact you are a high performer get out of hand. The purpose of this training program is to make the most of your training in a minimal amount of time to get the maximum results in order to still focus on business, well-being, and positive relationships.

THIS PROGRAM ISN'T FOR THE TRADITIONAL GYM RAT BUT SOMEONE WHO WANTS MORE THAN JUST THAT. YOU WANT THE HIGH PERFORMANCE LIFE AND YOUR BEST BODY.

If you are in a place where all those areas are doing well, and you have an extra hour to train a fourth day or fifth day, you can use that for a lagging body part. Men typically like to use their fourth training day for their chest or arms, while women like to use it for their glutes or legs.

I used my fourth day to build more rounded shoulders for competitions; it just depends on your personal or professional goals.

The most important part about training more than three days a week is recovery time. It makes no sense to train legs within two days of each other if they haven't yet recovered. Recovery is key when it comes to strength and getting the physique you want, just as much as recovery is needed mentally for you to kick ass as a high performer.

Just as you can't be a high performer without renewing your energy daily, you can't be training at a more advanced level without renewal or recovery. They are correlated.

ABS, CARDIO, CALVES

Abs can be done once or twice a week with training like any other muscle. While focusing on the major muscle groups like legs, back, and chest, your core is part of that.

Cardio is secondary to weight training unless you are specifically an endurance athlete. I have found when people want to put more energy to losing weight and getting healthier, they think the first thing they need to do is cut out meat and do insane cardio every day.

Cardio is not where the magic happens to get the high-performing physique you are after. You can use it to turn up the dial of your intensity for overall conditioning after the priority of weight training but never to replace unless it's part of your particular sport.

Calves are quite simple and I tag on a few sets at the end of leg day, and that's if I even remember.

PROFESSIONAL COMPETITORS

Yes, professional competitors can compete in shows using this program as a base, but you will need to hire a professional contest prep coach to manipulate macros. Every division looks for something different, so it's not a one size fits all in the professional world.

Like I said above, I used a fourth day to build up my shoulders, simply because the judges look for rounded shoulder caps and bigger size at the national level. Although I knew I'd compete against girls using drugs, I was okay knowing I was doing well without them, completely a fat burner- and drug-free.

As a competitor, it's most important to learn your own identity and lifestyle outside of being on stage. Competing at this level does not make you a high performer, but learning how to balance it all, including your overall well-being and relationships, for a long period of time does.

Many competitors expect that level-ten intensity out of themselves for years, while all the important things in life begin to fade. You are more than just counting macros and bringing your best package to the stage. It's just a sport. Your mind and body still need renewal and recovery; your relationships still need nurturing and managing; your career or business always has opportunities to grab hold of and invest into.

You can have all the trophies in the world, but when you get to the end of your life, none of it matters if you didn't learn how to live the High Performance life you were given in order to balance it. It's okay to dial back from a ten. It's okay to not freak out about calories and macros.

Working with professional athletes, the best ones are more than just what they do on the field, the court, or the stage. The best ones go beyond that. They adjust their dials, and the best ones like John Meadows kept marriage, family, and faith a bigger priority. Or Blayne, who commits to keto and intermittent fasting, is captain of the Men's National Soccer Team and is a devoted husband, father, and Christian serving his community and underprivileged families.

I saw how people got obsessed, and an idol over anything can destroy you, your life, your marriage, your family, and any future goals. I saw many people obsess over every calorie, every macro, with their faces in their phones. "Bailey, get out of doing shows.

You are a good person and it's going to ruin you," one earlier trainer of mine warned. It opened my eyes to be aware of the mentality he was concerned about, and that partly inspired me to write this book.

KEY TAKEAWAY

Now that you understand your very own dial and the fact that you can control it, set your own limits and grow. It's important to understand what level you are on. You aren't stuck there, but it helps to prevent injury and build on it to stay challenged and perform higher. Stay consistent with your three days per week. Moving from beginner to advanced allows you to train your mind to get the results you have always wanted.

With consistency, I continue to get stronger mentally and physically; so can you. I had to get inside my head to do it; you can get inside of yours. There is no waiting for others to push you or challenge you, but that's up to you and why I wrote this book.

HIGH-PERFORMANCE EXERCISE

You really need to paint this picture of what you want, visualize it, and feel the feels.

Decide what kind of high performer you want to be; visualize yourself, and explore how it would feel to live that. From your career, marriage, family, adventures, goals, health, and fitness.

With your life wheel, you can have that clarity of where you want to go, what to achieve, and who you want to be. While making goals for each area, you can be as specific as how fit and healthy you want to be at the same time as performing higher in the other nine areas.

Maybe you want to get in the best shape of your life, increase your muscle, decrease fat, and feel stronger and healthier than ever. And you want to do it while being deeply connected with your wife, happier with your work, being more present at home, and increasing your income.

Paint that picture for yourself and write it down.

Every Sunday, you evaluate the joy in each of those ten areas. You can achieve everything in the world, but if you don't have joy, then you don't have much at all. Or maybe you're so focused on one area like your career or health, that your marriage falls apart. This wheel is critical to having joy to move forward in every area of your life...not just one or two.

It's more than just owning a business and making big money. It's more than just losing the weight and having your dream body. It's more than just the next accomplishment; although those are all important, you need joy in the picture, too. You know it.

You not only have the ideas, the goals, the pictures, the inspiration, but the tools and tactics to get you there and to keep you there.

Be honest with yourself right now (and always) to avoid injury and to keep getting stronger AF.

1. Are you a beginner, intermediate, or advanced right now?
2. Based on your level above, list one to three things you need to be mindful of while training. For example, if you're a beginner, then maybe it's about using great form and only doing warm-up sets for each exercise until you acclimate. If intermediate, maybe it's blocking out distractions while training to get into

the zone, or being able to complete all the warm-up sets and working sets. If advanced, maybe it's learning how to use mind-muscle connection, or using bands to resist or assist your lifts.

3. On a scale from one to ten, where are you? If life is overwhelming, give yourself permission that it's okay to lower your dial. Do you need to lower your dial? Turn it up? If so, where do you need it to be right now in order to kick ass in every area of life and be strong AF? Only you have that dial to adjust...nobody else.

CONCLUSION

Now you have everything you need to know for getting fit in less time so you can be happy in every area of your life, too. You are kicking ass in every area of your life or at least working your way toward it, especially the areas that matter the most like treasuring your wife and kids.

And you deserve your Mr. Banks moment, too.

The most special transformation for Mr. Banks didn't occur until the end of *Mary Poppins* when he repaired the kite. His kids were so full of excitement and joy to see what he had done and to spend time laughing in the park while they learned to fly it together. He flew that kite with his kids and was completely present and joyful, not checking his watch. He finally realized he wasn't going to miss the important things anymore.

That can be you. You too can be successful and present like Mr. Banks. You can realize what is important and focus on that—and by following this book, you get the bonus of being jacked!

It took far too long for Mr. Banks to realize what matters most in life. He chased what he thought was success at the expense of his kids, wife, and joy. I don't want you to miss out, and I don't think you want to either.

It was a beautiful and magical movie. The unexpected thing for me was learning that it was partly inspired by a true story—without the animated dancing penguins, of course.

After writing this book, I watched *Saving Mr. Banks*, a movie that told about how Walt Disney wanted to turn the book *Mary Poppins* into the movie, but the author was extremely difficult to work with, to say the least.

She had a reason, though: she was Mr. Banks's daughter in real life and had a tragic childhood. She had fond memories of her dad, and it grieved her to think of remembering him in that way.

It took Walt Disney twenty years to convince the author to turn it into the movie, which he did by promising to redeem her dad. That's the reason Mr. Banks finally changes at the end and is able to fly a kite with his kids, all thanks to Mary Poppins.

You need to fly your kite and not wait twenty years to be convinced.

So let this book be the Mary Poppins to your Mr. Banks, where you find joy and purpose and treasure your family again, all while getting built and strong AF in every area of your life.

YOU CAN DO THIS, TOO

You can be Mr. Banks with a six pack, happy wife, and loving kids.

With only three days a week—and a spoonful of sugar to help the medicine go down—you can have a different mindset for the life-style, health, happiness, and body you've always wanted. You can be fit in only three days a week so those other areas don't suffer, all while keeping the important things the most important.

You truly can kick ass at life.

You are more than just a body. You are more than your career. You are a human being full of life, and you should live it to its fullest.

You can be like Greg who now thinks more clearly, keeping self-care and workouts a priority. He not only became leaner and stronger, but he's also more productive with his business and overall more successful.

Or if you need to, you can dial it back, like I did myself with my losses of 2020 or Blayne had to do after his brain injuries. I was still able to complete this book for you by dialing it back to what my mind and body needed most, while keeping God, marriage, and family first. Blayne took the time off to heal and came back stronger as the national team captain.

Or be like Billy who was at his lowest point in his life and then completely turned it around with these simple tips so he could focus more on a joy-filled life, becoming fitter and stronger than he was as a semi-pro soccer player.

Or think of John, who inspired the world, whom I learned from.

Whom the best from around the world learned from. He did it while keeping his faith and family a priority while owning a few businesses and coaching Olympians. Like he said at his Arnold Classic seminar, he wanted you to get that so bad.

They all desired that High Performance life deep down and made it their lifestyle. It wasn't a diet or a fad or just a sport. It was their whole life. And so much simpler than people realize.

They all became built, strong, and healthier while focusing on what matters most in life—and while learning to dream.

MY DAD LET GO OF HIS KITE

I wish I could have given Dad a copy of this book. He just worked so hard, as so many of us do. We work so hard but don't know how to be present and do what matters most.

He still did it with a smile and the gentlest of spirits. He was the one praying with terrified patients about to go into surgery or giving life advice to anyone who asked for his wisdom. Anyone who met him adored and remembered him.

The ALS advanced so much that at the age of fifty-eight, he couldn't speak, blink, or use his arms or legs. However, he was mentally all there, just trapped in his own body and wanting to do so much more. My brother and I held him up as he walked me down the aisle.

Eventually, ALS patients pass from respiratory failure because the muscles that help you breathe become paralyzed like the rest of the body and you suffocate. The day soon came when the hospice nurse told us he probably wouldn't live to see the next day.

The next day, we took him home from the hospital. We set up our parents' bed and the three oxygen generators that helped him breathe. This all was surely a gift to have one more moment with Dad and for him to be at peace at home.

"Could you read the scriptures where Jesus was washing the feet of the disciples for me?" My brother brought in a washbasin, removed Dad's socks, and gently washed his feet.

Trying not to choke on my own emotions, I read John 13:1: "Jesus knew that the hour had come for him to leave this world and go to the Father. Having loved his own who were in the world, he loved them to the end."

I remembered a dream I had about my dad almost fifteen years earlier. In it, he was fighting the gusty wind while attempting to fly a kite. He tried controlling it, but not until he finally let go did he actually have peace. In the dream, I could see he had the peace that surpassed all understanding. He wasn't fighting or frustrated anymore of working so hard but had an overwhelming amount of peace and the bluest of eyes.

I asked God what I was to do with that dream, so I prayed for Dad to experience such a peace whether it was in this life on earth or if that would be the peace he'd experience in heaven.

I never felt the timing of sharing that dream with him until almost fifteen years later, after my brother had washed his feet and prepared him to leave this world and go to the Father. Then I told him, "Dad, years ago, I believe God gave me a dream for you. In this dream, I saw you fighting the wind with this kite. When you let go and watched the kite freely fly away, the peace that was all over you was overwhelming and beautiful. You were free and covered in peace and joy, and your eyes were the bluest of blues...and I want you to have that kind of peace, Dad."

I tried describing this heavenly picture I had of this unexplainable peace and joy. But the words were just that—unexplainable.

"Dad, it's okay to let go of that kite and have that peace and freedom."

A dear friend shared that hearing is the last sense to go with the dying, so it was important to continue speaking sweet words to him. Singing the childhood songs he introduced us to, reading more of the *Jesus Calling* devotional, and reading scriptures. His pastors visited and prayed in his last few hours, and I read my daughter's *Bedtime Prayers*.

Mom was curled up next to Dad, holding his hand and reminding him of what an amazing husband, father, and friend he has been all these years. She thanked him for all the wonderful memories and vacations, and how he always put God and family first.

"It's okay to go home, Mike. We are all going to be okay. You gave us a wonderful life," Mom said in between her tears. Their marriage of thirty-eight years was a testament of love and selflessness. She was his full-time caretaker for these years. Although he couldn't move, his eyes always went to her.

It was only a few more breaths after finishing *Bedtime Prayers*, where we were prepping his next morphine dose, and there wasn't another breath.

"Mom, Dad's not breathing!"

It was the sentence I selfishly didn't want to speak but knew it was for his gain.

"I know," she said. "I felt it."

That was all I could hear Mom say with her head buried under her pillow still curled up next to him.

We were gathered around him, in awe of the peace over him. The kite was flying free. Peace that he had given God, his wife, kids, and church the best he ever could, and was in heaven singing beautifully once again in his pain-free body, in complete peace, joy, and freedom. He was probably dunking a basketball again, laughing with old friends, or perhaps sitting in awe of Jesus himself.

TIME IS PRECIOUS—GET STARTED!

Time is precious and sacred, and you don't get it back.

It's a gift and you should use it as such. Yes, you can be present with the people you love. You can get strong and built in much less time than you realize and kick ass in every area of life. Keep the energy up to keep doing it, and redefine success on your own terms.

So what should you do now?

Look at your schedule for when you want to fit in one hour at the gym three days a week. It doesn't need to be more than that. Simplify your nutrition and training according to your own dial and adjust it as needed. After your first week, reevaluate to see if you need to turn up the dial or maybe even dial it back.

I've included a few workouts just to get you started for your very first week, but you don't want to do the same thing every week. Get more free tools we talked about in this book and more training at http://www.threedaysstrongaf.com/.

By simplifying your training and nutrition that is laid out in this book, you can have the health and fitness you've always desired while also performing higher in all the other areas, too.

Enjoy your new life with *Three Days Strong AF*.

With love,

Your Mary Poppins

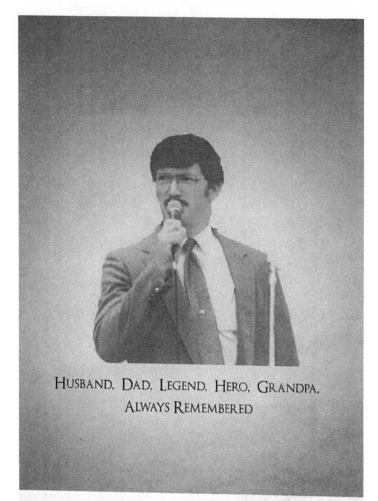

HUSBAND, DAD, LEGEND, HERO, GRANDPA,
ALWAYS REMEMBERED

MICHAEL E. BAILEY, SR.

■ ■ ■

October 23, 1954 - July 27, 2017

APPENDIX

TRAINING WORKOUTS TO MAXIMIZE RESULTS AND SIMPLIFY YOUR LIFE

First, you will need a fully equipped gym. One that has free weights, leg press, machines, cable machines, squat rack, Smith machine, dead lifts, bench that lies flat, inclined, and declined. For the advanced readers, use bands and chains to attach to bench press, dead lift, and squats.

Second, get your nutrition according to your dial. Whether you customize your meal plan by using your hand to measure, or you follow one of the examples I've provided in Chapter 5. Time your nutrition so the most important meals take place around training, for pre-workout meal, intra-workout meal, and post-workout meal.

Third, choose just three days you can spend one hour in the gym. You'll need to hit the largest muscle groups for the maximum results, and I have examples for you below. Once you have adjusted to three hours in the gym, then introduce your abs, calves, and

HIIT to after training or on off days. You'll have back day, chest day, and leg day. Add a fourth day if you want.

Fourth, mentally prepare yourself before lifting. Watch video tutorials. Execute it in your mind before getting to the gym. Tap into the power of mind-muscle connection where you get even greater results. Walk in with the confidence of how to do each workout whether you are a beginner or advanced. Be smart, not injured. Visualization is mental practice professional athletes do, and you can do it, too.

Fifth, grow as an overall high performer, not just in the gym. Don't just improve your health and body, but improve the joy in your marriage, family, relationships, adventures, mission/work, finances, adventure, hobby, spirituality, and emotions. Take the hammer to the rock and shine. See what you are made of and enjoy it. You really can have health and true joy, and the important things should never be on the back burner.

Why is this different than other training programs you can get? Well, one more reason is that this guide teaches you mind-muscle control. Look up workouts and most will simply tell you four sets of this and four sets of that. Here, we are tapping into mind-muscle control to activate the muscle you are working and building confidence and results even faster.

Below is a few weeks of training examples. Adjust to your level of experience. If you are a beginner, maybe you can only use your own body weight until you gain strength and mobility. If advanced and you've been training for a while, you can even add chains and resistive and assistive bands to the squats, dead lifts, and bench press.

TRAINING DAY EXAMPLES
WEEK ONE
Leg Day
Leg Press

While lowering the leg press, keep your knees out while many have the tendency to turn knees in. Have a stable stance, lower to where you begin to feel it in your hips. Don't be afraid to lower it deep to get your hips into it. Do 2–3 warm-up sets of 12. Keep adding a little bit of weight for each set until you find a pretty challenging weight. Do 3 sets of 12 with that. Drive through your heels, and make sure your knees and toes are in the same direction. After last set, do 2 sets of 15–20 calf raises on the leg press. (Once a week, add a few minutes of calves at the end of leg day to simplify your training.)

Rest 45–60 seconds between sets.

Barbell Squat

Feet slightly wider than shoulder-width apart, toes slightly pointed out, and knees in the same direction. Lower down in a 3-second count like you are sitting in a chair, and get your thighs to parallel. At that point, squeeze your butt, then blast up. Keep your core engaged and tight, chest up. Don't bend over with the bar, but shoot straight up to protect your back. The squat is never mastered, but every leg day is a chance to make it better than the rep before! Do 1–2 warm-ups of 10 until you feel warmed up, then 3 sets of 10. The warm-ups are just as important as the actual working sets so make sure you feel your blood pumping.

Seated Leg Curls

Squeeze hamstrings hard, then 3-second release for 10 reps. Then grab a heavy dumbbell to superset with 20 plié dumbbell squats. Keep core tight, shoulders back, chest up, and when you get to the bottom, squeeze your glutes to come back up. Do 3 rounds.

Leg Extension

1 warm-up set of 12. Squeeze quads for 2 seconds at the top. 3 times 12.

Note: Anytime the foot is planted, such as when doing squats, dead lifts, and leg press, it's important to use a three-point stance in your feet, and not drive through your heels as most trainers suggest.

Doctor of physical therapy Corey Southers explained, "While it has long been taught in many circles to always 'push from the heels' with certain activities, i.e., squats and leg press most notably, this is not necessarily the best practice when trying to get the best force production out of the nervous system. The midline and the pelvis (read the abs, the back, and the glutes) get a great deal of input from the pressure coming through the entire foot. Because of that, it is very important to approach any activity where the foot is planted with the notion of forming a 'tripod' with the foot—big toe knuckle, little toe knuckle, and heel should all be making uniform contact, and you should be aiming to produce equal force throughout all three of those points for the best force production and muscle recruitment throughout the entire chain. Let's get away from the notion of only pushing through one part of the foot, and let's respect the fact that we have a FULL foot for a reason."

Chest and Triceps

Rest 45–60 seconds between sets.

Dumbbell Bench Press

Do 2–3 sets of 12 to warm up. Slowly increase in weight every set. Once you are warmed up, then you do your 3 sets of 12. Grab two dumbbells not too terribly heavy for your first week. Perfect form is what we want. I like a small arch in my lower back when training chest because it helps develop more power when you will go heavy eventually. But for now, small arch, feet firm on the ground, and lower dumbbells next to your armpits where you feel them stretching. When you feel a good stretch, squeeze your pecs together and bring the weights back up squeezing them together.

Dumbbell Incline Press

Use the same concept as the last exercise to stretch your pecs and shoulders. But be sure to squeeze the hell out of your pecs. Do 1–2 warm-up sets of 12, then your 3 x 12. Increase weight to keep it difficult but with no injuries.

Chest Fly

Grab two lighter dumbbells and lie on a flat bench. Keep slight bend in elbows and lower at 3–5 seconds past until you feel the stretch in your pecs. Then initiate the movement at your pecs to bring the weights together slowly. Focus on the stretch here for 10–12 reps. Superset with 10 push-ups. After the 10 wide push-ups, rest 45–60 seconds and repeat for 3 total rounds.

Three Rounds to Finish Your Triceps

Superset from bench dips, to the double tricep kickback, to the rope pushdowns, and THEN rest about 60–90 seconds. On the double tricep kickback, have your side toward the mirror so you can watch your triceps work. Kick back, but then squeeze the dumbbell another inch or two higher to really make sure you are hitting the triceps. Keep core engaged with all of these.

- Bench dips x 10
- Double tricep kickback with dumbbells x 15
- Rope pushdown x 20
- Repeat 3 times.

After chest days and back days, these are great times to do a little cardio and then to also cool down and stretch.

Back and Biceps
Lat Pull Down

Wide grip, chest up, and an arch in your lower back to engage your lats even more. It's too easy to be lazy on this machine, but not you. Make your mind connect with your body and be intentional with every movement. Bring the bar down to your chest, keeping your core tight and hold for one second. Release in a controlled manner, and when the bar is at the top, let your shoulder blades relax out and stretch out a little bit. After they stretch, mentally visualize your lats right around your shoulder blade area initiating the movement and squeeze back down. Visualize every rep. And make each rep more perfect than the rep before. Do 2 sets of 12 to warm up like this and slowly add a little more weight that makes you work. Then 3 x 12.

Barbell Bent-over Row

You can use a Smith machine for this one. Feet shoulder-width apart, knees slightly bent. Bend at the hip over the bar with your lower back slightly arched to engage your core. With an overhand grip on the bar, bring the bar to touch your lower ribs. Squeeze it there for 2 seconds engaging your core and your back, then slowly lower down. Do 1 warm-up set of 10, then 3 sets of 10.

Cable Seated Rows

Sit on your "sit bones" as they say in yoga. Straighten your legs so when you bend at your hips (and never at your back), you are also getting a little hamstring stretch. Allow your shoulder blades to stretch out, and while keeping an arch in your lower back, drive your elbows to the wall behind you and squeeze your shoulder blades down and back. Although usually you are to keep a slight bend in your knees as most trainers explain, we are looking to add a simple stretch by keeping your legs straight and bend at the hips. Three sets of 12.

One-Arm Dumbbell Row

Do 1 set of 12 to warm up, then 3 sets of 12. Do 12 on the right, 12 on the left. Time your rest 45–60 seconds, then repeat. Use your hands as hooks for the weight, and mindfully keep all the tension in your lats. As you are lowering the dumbbell, feel your shoulder blade stretch out a little bit. Where you feel that stretch, that's where you want to squeeze to bring the dumbbell back up.

Biceps

Now that your back is all pumped, it also had your biceps warmed up, so we are just going to go ahead and get a quick bicep workout in. You don't need to rest as long with your arms as you do for larger muscle groups, so keep the rest minimal to 30–45 seconds, if that.

Superset 4 rounds.

One-Arm Preacher Curl

Do 4 sets of 10. Do a set of 10 with each side, then superset with the EZ bar bicep curl for 8. Rest minimally and do this 4 times.

EZ Bar Bicep Curl

Do 4 sets of 8; squeeze really hard at the top.

Shoulder Workout

To get accustomed to your first week and managing the time, I intentionally left shoulders out of the first week chest day. Just so you can find your rhythm in time management and start adding shoulders into the end of your chest workouts. However, if you have time for a fourth training day and would like a day to train your shoulders separately, here's a great workout that I love.

Machine Shoulder Press

Warm up 2 sets: Do 15 half reps of the top half of the movement, then 15 half reps of the bottom half, and then 15 full reps (45 is one warm-up set).

- After warm-up, go a little heavier where you are challenged but not injuring your shoulder joints. Do heavier for 10, then lighten the weight without a rest and do 10 more as a drop set. After 20 reps, then rest 60–90 seconds. Do 4 rounds.

Smith Machine Shoulder Press

Drag a bench to sit under the Smith machine bar. Press overhead for 15, then walk over to the cable rope for 20 face pulls. Rest 60–90 seconds. Do 4 rounds.

Dumbbell Lateral Raises

With slightly bent elbows, go heavier than what you normally do with straight-armed dumbbell lateral raises. Do heavier bent elbows for 10, then without rest, grab lighter dumbbells for strict form and straight elbows for 10 more. Rest 60–90 seconds. Do 4 rounds.

- Strict-Form Lateral Raises: Straight arms but just a slight bend in the elbow.

Reverse Pec Deck Flies

Sit facing the pec deck machine. This is great for your rear deltoids. Do 20, and then grab dumbbells for front raises for the front of your shoulders. With the front raises, bring the dumbbell to right above eye level and lower slowly for 3 seconds. Do 20 of those, then rest 60–90 seconds. Do 4 rounds.

WEEK TWO

Leg Day

Warm-up, stretch, and resting is only between the sets for 45–60 seconds.

Barbell Good Mornings

Focus on feeling the stretch in the hamstrings, pushing hips back. No injuries, so be smart and safe, perfecting each rep BETTER than the rep before it. 4 sets of 12.

Seated Leg Curls

Do 1–2 warm-up sets (do more if you need it) then 12, 10, 8, drop set for 12. Pyramid up in weight on those leg curls. Build up to a tough weight for 12, rest 45–60 seconds, then add more weight for 10. Rest, then add more weight for 8. For the last 12 on the leg curl, take off a plate and make the most of it. Be stretching between sets.

Leg Press

Warm up with sets of 10 and keep adding weight until you find a struggling weight, then use that for 3 more sets of 10. Toes slightly wider than shoulder-width apart, toes slightly pointed out and knees in same direction. For those 3 sets, superset with lighter dumbbell stiff-leg dead lifts to get more stretching for your hamstrings. Rest, repeat for 3 rounds.

Dumbbell Stiff-Leg Dead Lift

Except these dead lifts aren't supposed to be too heavy. Keep your hips back, and as you lower the bar, make the main focus the stretch in your hamstrings. Once you feel that stretch, squeeze the hell out of your glutes to bring it back to the top. Bend at hips, NOT at your back! Really push those hips back. Repeat. 3 rounds of 10.

Bench Step-ups

Do 12 on the right and left side, then superset with 12 to 15 reverse lunges. Build that booty! Rest, then do 2 more rounds.

Leg Extension

Finish off your quads. Find a moderate to heavy weight and go until failure squeezing your quads hard each time. If you are going too fast, add more weight and control your pace. It doesn't do you any good to move fast through the movements.

Chest, Shoulders, and Triceps
Hammer Strength Incline Press

Do 2–3 warm-up sets. 12, 10, 8, 12. Add each time and find something you struggle for 12 reps. Rest 90 seconds, then add a little more for 10 more reps. Rest 90 seconds and add a little more weight for 8. Then do the same weight you did for 12 for your last 10 reps. Targeting upper chest, and keep feet on the ground. Hands are slightly wider than shoulder-width to keep the target on the chest. Keep arch in lower back, chest up. If you keep your back flat, you are using more of your front delts than your chest, so get that arch that feels comfortable for you.

Barbell Bench Press

Do 2–3 warm-up sets as needed. Rest. Pause your working sets by slowly lowering the weight to chest, and let it rest there for 2 seconds, then drive up without locking elbows. I use a slight arch in my lower back with feet firm on the ground. 3 sets of 6.

Pec Deck Machine

Do 3 sets of 10, and each set superset with 10 wide push-ups. After the push-ups, then rest 60–90 seconds. Keep elbows slightly bent and focus on feeling your chest squeezing as you bring the handles closer together.

Seated Dumbbell Rear Lateral Raises

30, 25, 20, then 15 with up to 2-minute rest between sets.

Mountain Dog Six Ways

These are shoulder burners. John Meadows introduced me to these. Grab light dumbbells. Hold them at your sides, then raise them laterally to shoulder height. From there, bring them together in front of you to touch, then up over your head, back down to front, then down to shoulder height again, then down to your side for one rep. These really do burn! 3 sets of 7 or 8.

Finish up with some triceps. Make sure you are extending your triceps like an extra half inch just to be sure you're getting the different tricep heads and then squeeze for a solid second or two.

Rope Pushdowns, Then Superset with EZ Bar Skull Crushers

Do 15 pushdowns with really squeezing your triceps, then grab the EZ bar for 10 more skull crushers. See if you can stretch your triceps a little bit as you lower the bar. Don't flare out your elbows. Do this for 3 rounds, but if you think you can squeeze out 4, THEN GO FOR IT!!

Superset 3 rounds.

Rope Pushdowns 3 x 15

EZ Bar Skull Crushers 3 x 10

Back and Biceps

Focus on feeling your shoulder blade relax on the dumbbell row, lat pull down, and cable row before engaging movement in lats. Each movement is intentional.

Intention.

A word full of action to make the most out of life, the most out of this work, the most of every single rep. Make the most, and be intentional. Meditate on that one.

Rest about 45–60 seconds.

Dumbbell One-Arm Row

Do 2–3 warm-up sets of 12 to get up to a difficult weight. Then add weight each set for 12, 10, 8. Allow shoulder blade to relax when dumbbell is coming close to the ground, then engage your lat to initiate movement driving elbow back. Feel your back, not your arms. Arms are only helpers in back exercises.

Dumbbell Lying Pullover

Heavier dumbbell and lie on back on a flat bench, keep arms straight and bring the dumbbell over and behind your head until you feel your lats stretching right below/behind your armpits. When you feel THAT stretch, engage that exact spot to initiate bringing the dumbbell back up over your forehead. Warm up 1–2 sets of 12 until you feel blood pumping, then do 3 x 12.

One-Arm Cable Rows

With left foot up on pad, grab handle with right arm. Drive elbow to back wall and squeeze back an extra inch or two than what you could if you were using two hands. Release and allow shoulder blade to stretch out, then drive elbow back again. Remember to keep the focus in your back, not your arms. 3 sets of 10.

Close-Grip Lat Pull Downs

Keep small arch in lower back and chest up. Here, you are using the attachment where your hands are facing each other. Squeeze shoulder blades down and back for 3 sets of 12. After each set, superset with pull-ups until failure. Use a pull-up assist machine, or rig rubber band up to do an assisted pull up. But do as many as you can, then rest 45–60. Do this 3 times.

Now that your biceps are warmed up, let's squeeze out another few sets to get your biceps in. If you don't like doing biceps and triceps at the end of your workouts, you can train arms on a whole separate day. Do what works best for you. I personally prefer not to live in the gym, but to each their own!

Incline Dumbbell Curl

Do 3 sets of 12. Set up the bench about a 45-degree angle, and the angle allows your long head of your biceps to stretch. You can grab two dumbbells to do both arms at the same time and activate those biceps at every curl.

EZ Bar Bicep Curl

Do 3 sets of 10. Knees and elbows are kept soft. Squeeze biceps at the top of the movement, and slowly lower for 2–3 seconds.

ADVANCED WORKOUTS
Leg Day

Another variation of the traditional squat is the box squat. In this movement, you squat until you are sitting on a platform or box. This is typically placed just at or above parallel. It is essential that you transfer all weight to the platform, pause, and then drive upward. This technique works the weakest range of motion by forcing you to have a "cold start" from the bottom, similar if using chains or bands to your lifts. Squeeze the glutes to drive upward and keep the torso as vertical as possible (many people make the mistake of leaning forward before driving up from the platform, and this may lead to injury). If you don't have a box at the gym, grab a bench to sit back on.

You want it to be about knee level or even below. From the point of sitting on the box or bench to standing up and completing the exercise, you want the barbell to be in one direct vertical line, not swaying back and forth. It is easy to sway as you sit and come up from the box/bench, so focus on taking that bar directly to the ceiling without bending forward. This really targets glutes and hamstrings. Do 2–3 warm-up sets, increasing weight and watch that knees aren't going over the toes. Complete with 3 sets of 20.

Plié Squat

Increase weight of dumbbell each set, but instead of coming all the way up, do only to one-fourth of a rep at the bottom. So sink low where you feel your hips stretching and glutes working, squeeze them hard, and only come up one-fourth of the way, engaging glutes and core the entire time. Remember to keep shoulders back and chest up and out. Don't lean forward. 3 x 15.

Seated Leg Curls

One thing I love about training is focusing on the blood pumping into the muscle to get it working. Visualize the muscle. Feel the blood feeding that area and really focus on each rep. Do 10, 8, and 6 increasing weight each time.

Superset for 3 rounds:

1. **Leg press** with feet shoulder-width apart, toes pointed out, knees in the same direction to keep things in alignment and train more of the front of your quads. Drive through the three points on your feet. Don't allow knees to lock out, yet squeeze the front of your quads hard to get shape and strength. *Keep knees out, same direction as toes, and don't let those knees buckle. On the last rep, walk platform up ready for your calf raises. Need a bend in knees for the calves. Superset directly into leg extension. 3 x 12 for leg press.
2. **Calf raises** on the leg press for 15–20 reps.

3. **Leg extensions** by SQUEEZING the hell out of your quads. Keep constant tension on the quads. 3 x 12.

Then rest 45–60 seconds between rounds.

Chest, Shoulders, and Triceps

Joint Care. The biggest part of the warm-ups is to get the blood moving to nourish the muscles and to prevent injuries. Weight training in itself not only helps you get a winning physique and burning fat faster than any other method (when done correctly), but it's great for strengthening your joints. Don't skip warm-ups or get sloppy on your form because you'll end up damaging your joints and causing injury. Always be smart while challenging yourself.

Pec Deck Machine

Do 2 sets of 20 for a warm-up, then find a good weight for 12. Count 3 seconds as you lower, then squeeze for 1 second. Rest for 2 minutes if you need to, then add a little more weight. It's going to be tough to start this way, so talk yourself up, get in your head. 3 x 12.

Dumbbell Press with a Twist

Do this on a flat bench, twisting at the top. Don't forget to stretch your pecs on the way down and then drive up. It's okay to have an arch in your lower back and to engage your core and lats to drive up more weight. Do 1–2 warm-up sets. Do a third. Whatever it takes to make sure your joints are properly warmed up, then follow with 12, 10, 8, increasing weight each round. Really challenge yourself. If you are getting sloppy, you only end up slowing down any progress you want to see and feel, not to mention you're at risk of injury. Be mindful of every single rep.

Barbell Bench Press on Incline Bench

This won't take much weight; you should be tired by now. Rest pause on your chest. Lower bar slowly for 3 seconds to chest and let it rest there for 2 seconds and then drive up hard without locking out elbows. 3 sets of 6.

John Meadows-Style Side Laterals

Do 12 solid reps, lowering 3 seconds. Then second set, go up in weight a little for 10 more. Go up again if you can and do 8 reps. Rest only 10 seconds, then do 4 reps, then rest 5 seconds, and do 2 more. Set your mind and drill this one. 12, 10, 8, 4, 2.

Front Raise with Dumbbells

Lower slowly. Have control over each rep. Don't take above eye level. 3 x 12.

Superset tricep for 3 rounds.

Standing Cable Tricep Pushdown Bar

Find a good weight for 3 sets of 12, and superset with 8–12 bench dips. Grab a plate to put on your lap to make it harder for the dips. If it's still too easy, then grab two plates. It's easier to have a partner put them there, but it can be done on your own, too.

Back and Biceps
Smith Machine Bent-over Row

Set the pins a little below the knee because you are going to set the bar down for rest pauses. First do 2–3 warm-up sets, squeezing the bar against your upper abs while keeping your back flat and at a 45-degree angle over the bar. Be sure you are using your lats to drive up the bar. Add weight each time and be explosive as you get warmed up. After a few warm-up sets, get to a weight that you struggle with 8 and do 2 sets of 8. Each rep, set the bar down on the pins, then drive back up. Add more weight and do 2 sets of 6 rest pauses. 4 x 8, 8, 6, 6.

Cable Rows

Multitask on this one. Most trainers have you bend your knees, but keep them straight so you can work in hamstring stretches at each rep. Don't bend at your back, but bend at your hips to stretch your hamstrings. Reach forward as far as you can, then bring a good arch in your lower back to focus the movement in your lats HEAVILY. Really stretch them. Sit up straight, arch chest up and out, and squeeze shoulder blades down and back. Do this right and it will feel good! Pyramid up in weight each time. 10, 8, 6.

*As you stretch forward, allow your shoulder blades to also stretch forward. In a fluid movement, initiate FIRST movement in your lats, then drive elbows to the wall behind you flexing and squeezing your upper back. Hold, and slowly release to your stretch position again.

Dumbbell Pullover for Lats

Focus on feeling the stretch in your lats for the dumbbell pullover.

That stretch is the indicator to bring the weight back up over to your chest. Use slow and controlled movements while paying close attention to shoulder joints. Ease the weight behind and over your head until you feel a stretch in the lats just below your shoulders. Initiate pulling the weight back over your head at that very spot. Visualize that muscle contracting all the way until you bring the weight above your chest. This hits triceps and chest as well, but keep the focus on pushing weight while stretching your lats in this movement. 3 x 12.

Partial Pull-ups

Only come about one-third of the way up. Relax your shoulder blades at the bottom and stretch, and come up a few inches.

Superset biceps for 3 rounds.

EZ Bar Reverse Curl

Palms face down on EZ bar to target the brachialis and brachioradialis in the arms. 3 x 8.

Standing Dumbbell Curls

Shoulders back, and keep elbows glued into your sides. Squeeze biceps hard as dumbbells come toward your shoulders, and lower for 3 seconds. Remember to exhale on the more difficult part of the exercise, such as curling the dumbbell.

EZ Bar Bicep Curl

3 x 8. Activate your core, chest up, shoulders back, and elbows at sides just like the dumbbell curls you just did.